JUDYLAINE FINE

Afraid to Ask

For all the teenagers, mothers, and fathers
who have had the courage to share their pain . . .
and for Harold S. Fine who has always shown courage.

Text copyright © 1984, 1986 by Judylaine Fine.
Illustrations copyright © 1984 by Dorothy Irwin.
Cover photograph copyright Mieke Maas/Image Bank Canada.
First published in Canada in 1984 by Kids Can Press.
All rights reserved. No part of this book may be reproduced or utilized in any form or by any means,
electronic or mechanical, including photocopying, recording or by any information storage and
retrieval system, without permission in writing from the Publisher. Inquiries should be addressed
to Lothrop, Lee & Shepard Books, a division of William Morrow & Company, Inc.,
105 Madison Avenue, New York, New York 10016.
Printed in the United States of America.   First U.S. Edition 1986.
First Beech Tree edition, 1991
1 3 5 7 9 10 8 6 4 2

Library of Congress Cataloging in Publication Data
Fine, Judylaine.   Afraid to ask.
Bibliography: p. Includes index. Summary: Describes the various types of cancer and discusses,
through case histories, the physical and emotional problems involved in having or
knowing someone who has cancer.
1. Cancer—Juvenile literature. 2. Tumors in children—Juvenile literature. [I. Cancer] I. Title.
RC263.F526 1986   616.99'4   85-28386
ISBN 0-688-06196-6 (pbk.)
Medical illustrations by Dorothy Irwin.

Contents

Acknowledgments

I can't adequately express my gratitude to the people who helped make this book possible. By answering my thousands of questions and wading through my explanations with fine-tooth combs, these dedicated people have shattered my impression that people in the health care professions are unwilling to share their time.

Dr. Richard Hasselback, senior medical oncologist at the Princess Margaret Hospital in Toronto, read and commented on the manuscript on three separate occasions. In a sense he is the godfather of *Afraid to Ask*.

The following people read and commented on the manuscript, and I am especially indebted to them: Alan Bernstein, Ph.D., molecular geneticist, Ontario Cancer Institute; Dr. Saul Levine, chief of psychiatry, Sunnybrook Hospital, Toronto; Dr. Anthony Miller, director, epidemiology unit, National Cancer Institute of Canada; Cheryl Moyer, national director of public education, Canadian Cancer Society; David Nostbakken, Ph.D., president, International Liaison Committee for Smoking and Health, and project director, Smoking Control Program for the Continent of Africa; Dr. Harry Schachter, head, research division, department of biochemistry, Hospital for Sick Children, Toronto.

I am grateful to the following people who granted me interviews: Bill Adair, national director of service to patients, Canadian Cancer Society; David Adams, M.S.W., director of social work services, McMaster University Medical Centre, Hamilton, Ontario; Margaret Arnold, Cansurmount Convener, Metropolitan Toronto, Canadian Cancer Society; Dr. Michael Baker, chief of oncology, Toronto General Hospital; Dr. Dee Burton, director of adult education, American Cancer Society; Marilyn Deachman, psychosocial liaison nurse, Princess Margaret Hospital; Dr. Barry DeVebber, director of hematology oncology, Victoria Hospital, London, Ontario; Dr. Hans Dosch, associate professor of pediatrics, division of immunology and rheumatology, department of pediatrics, Hospital for Sick Children, Toronto; Gerrit DeBoer, Ph.D., head, department of biostatistics, Ontario Cancer Institute; Stephen Fleming, Ph.D., associate professor of psychology, York University, Toronto; Dr. Erwin Gelfand, chief, division of immunology and rheumatology, department of pediatrics, Hospital for Sick Children, Toronto; Dr. Mark Greenberg, senior oncologist, division of hematology oncology, department of pediatrics, Hospital for Sick Children, Toronto; Zsolt Harsanyi, Ph.D., executive director, Porton International Ltd., New York; Joseph Hoffman, program director, Project D.A.R.E., South River, Ontario; Gabriel Lam, Ph.D., research biophysicist, Medical Biophysics Unit, B.C. Cancer Research Centre; Gordon Lang, bereavement counsellor, Victoria Hospital, London, Ontario; Dr. Dorothy Ley, executive director, The Palliative Care Foundation of Canada; The Reverend Pam McGee, director of chaplaincy services, The Wellesley and Princess Margaret Hospitals, Toronto; Marilyn MacKenzie, former head nurse, department of hematology oncology, Hospital for Sick Children; John Mahoney, president, National Hospice Organization, Washington, D.C.; Dr. Ed Pakes, senior psychiatrist, Hospital for Sick Children; Dr. Ralph Pohlman, consulting psychiatrist, Sunnybrook Hospital, Toronto; Peter Scholefield, Ph.D., executive director, National Cancer Institute of Canada; Dr. Michel Silberfeld, staff psychiatrist, Princess Margaret Hospital; Dr. Paul R. Torrens, professor of Health Services Administration, School of Public Health, University of California at Los Angeles; Mary Vachon, Ph.D., research scientist, Clark Institute of Psychiatry, Toronto.

I would also like to thank the American Cancer Society and the Canadian Cancer Society for generously providing me with material on many specific types of cancer.

Introduction

Two decades ago, the word "cancer" was rarely spoken. The disease was prevalent but not discussed. Many doctors avoided answering any questions that family members of cancer patients might have had about the disease. And, in fact, most of us never dared to ask.

Things have changed. Today, many doctors realize that families want to know the truth about cancer. The trouble is that while they want to satisfy these needs, knowing what to say, and how best to say it, is very difficult. In some instances, their own knowledge is lacking. In other instances, there simply are no answers; even the scientists are asking the same questions as you.

While scientists have learned what cancer is, for example, they still don't know many of the details that occur when a normal cell changes into a cancer cell. While they are aware of some of the factors that can increase a person's risk of developing cancer, they don't know exactly why one person gets the disease while another person does not.

Doctors know that almost half the people who get cancer will beat it. But they don't know for sure who will be in which half. This means they don't know for certain what will happen to the person about whom you are concerned.

In an attempt to protect people from emotional pain, many doctors leave facts unsaid. I have written this book because I believe very strongly that you are entitled to as much information about cancer as you need. *Afraid to Ask* tries to answer as many questions as possible, as directly as possible.

The first chapter explains what cancer is. If you are fascinated by scientific details, you will find them here. When I first began to do the research for this book, the science of cancer wasn't my main interest. Then I met Dr. Harry Schachter, a biochemist at the Hospital for Sick Children in Toronto, and I became intrigued. I wouldn't be surprised if the same thing happens to you.

But if understanding what cancer really is doesn't interest you as much as knowing who gets the disease, or how doctors treat it, go right to the chapter you feel a need to understand. If knowing about a particular type of cancer is what you are after, turn to the last section of the book. I have organized *Afraid to Ask* in such a way that it is not essential to start at the first page.

As for the questions for which there are still no answers, researchers are pressing ahead. Each day, it seems, more and more clues that could eventually lead to a cure for cancer are emerging. Scientists have never been more hopeful than they are today.

In the meantime, until these remaining mysteries can be solved, you will know at least that other people are asking too. Every year, over a million North Americans are diagnosed with cancer. You are not alone in what you are going through.

AFRAID TO ASK

PART I
Afraid to Ask

CHAPTER ONE
What Is Cancer?

"MY mother has had cancer. If I could only wrap my brain around what cancer is, I think somehow I'd be able to handle it better."

Jenny was sixteen when I met her. She had already been through a two-year battle with breast cancer—her mother's. Things were looking fairly hopeful by the time I talked to her. But those two years had been awful. First there had been surgery. Then grueling treatments with radiation and chemicals—chemotherapy, they call it—that left Jenny wondering how a treatment with such terrible side effects could possibly *cure* someone of a disease.

Jenny had read everything about cancer she could get her hands on: pamphlets; newspaper clippings; magazine articles. And yet, she still sensed that she didn't have a handle on what was going on.

"I know that every year more than a million North Americans get cancer," she told me. "I mean, I've read that. I've read that and a bunch of other figures a thousand times. But how does cancer start? Why can't doctors always cure it? What does it look like? Why does it start in one place and end up in another? I must have asked two dozen people these questions—doctors, teachers, social workers—but no one has ever given me any answers that really make sense."

A lot of things about cancer hadn't made much sense to

me either. But I had been lucky. When I had put out the word that I was working on this book, many professionals agreed to be interviewed. Everyone was excited that a book on cancer was being written for the family members of cancer patients—both teenagers and adults.

The week before I met Jenny, my understanding of cancer had suddenly increased by leaps and bounds. Someone had suggested I speak to Dr. Harry Schachter, a cancer researcher at Toronto's Hospital for Sick Children.

Dr. Schachter's down-to-earth explanations boomed across the room. "The trouble is, we don't really understand the *basics* of cancer. No one knows for certain why cancer starts.

"Why does a normal cell that's doing what it's supposed to do *stop* doing what it's supposed to be doing and become cancerous? What makes a cancer cell—unlike a normal cell—able to break off from the organ where it belongs?"

Dr. Schachter paused a moment for emphasis. "Did you know that a cancerous liver cell can move from the liver to set up shop in another organ—say the lung—where it grows into a second cancer tumor? Any *normal* liver cell would be dead in no time if it somehow got detached from its liver and found its way to a lung. The body doesn't allow normal liver cells to live in lungs. It doesn't let them live anywhere except in livers!

"The thing is, until we figure out the answers to all these questions, the cure for cancer will remain out of reach. And no one can say for sure when researchers will discover these answers."

There are many things about cancer that scientists do know. They know what cancer looks like, for example. Often they know how to treat it successfully—if it has been detected at an early stage. The trouble is, by the time a lot of cancers are discovered, they have had time to grow into hard, gritty tumors, at least the size of a pea. Frequently the first or primary tumor has already "shed" some of its cells, and they have traveled to other parts of the body to grow into secondary tumors. In that case there is more than one tumor to treat.

Some types of cancer grow in clusters that look, to the naked eye, like cauliflowers. Other kinds look more like the flesh of sliced fish. Still others, breast cancer for example, have fingers that radiate haphazardly like crabgrass into nearby tissue. In fact, the word "cancer" means crab, the animal with claws that radiate from the main part of its body.

But if you were to take a paper-thin slice of a cancer tumor and slap it between two pieces of glass under a microscope, what you'd see might surprise you. Many researchers have used the word "majestic" to describe how magnified cancer cells look. One physician, John MacDonald, died of lung cancer not long after he wrote *When Cancer Strikes*. He described cancer cells seen under a microscope as "a forest fire . . . a flock of birds frightened from their destined path . . . scattered in disarray." To me they look like the swirls of a multicolored marble cake before it has been baked.

While there are different descriptions of how cancer cells look, no one disagrees about how they perform. Cancer cells no longer do the job they are supposed to be doing. What's worse, they no longer act in the orderly way that cells in our bodies normally act. Instead, cancer cells divide like crazy, without rhyme or reason, without any regard for the rest of the body's needs. They may be liver cells in a liver that doesn't need any new cells and yet they continue to reproduce. They may be liver cells that have detached themselves from their liver and are living in a lung, or in a brain, or anywhere. As Dr. Schachter explained, a normal liver cell that had somehow broken off from its liver would never be allowed by the body to set up shop in another organ. Somehow, cancer cells can.

But the only way to grasp the mystery of cancer is to begin with the basics. Until you have an understanding of how cells are supposed to work, it's impossible to really understand what happens when things go wrong.

How Cancer Cells Work
To begin with, cancer is not a single disease. There are

more than one hundred different kinds of cancer. Scientists have been able to show that different things—certain chemicals, radiation, and some viruses—can cause cancer. Basically, cancer is a disturbance in cell physiology—the mechanics of how a cell works.

How cells work is an extremely complicated matter. They are not, for example, like cars. When your car isn't running properly, you take it to a mechanic. He knows where every bolt goes, what every piston does, and what makes the car's engine work. It's relatively easy to fix something when you understand its mechanics.

Unfortunately, how normal cells work is not yet understood, not by a long shot. In the past ten years, scientists have unraveled a great number of mysteries, but many basic questions still remain unanswered.

Scientists don't understand, for example, how each cell knows what its particular job is. They don't understand how some of the cells in the liver know that their job is to produce proteins that can purify blood. Or how these same liver cells also know when it's time to reproduce by dividing into two new liver cells to replace ones that have died. Scientists also have very little idea how these cells know that it's time to *stop* reproducing when there is just the right number of new liver cells.

Until these riddles are solved, scientists won't be able to explain why cancer cells stop following the rules that govern all normal cells.

But let's go back to the beginning. Imagine that millions of years ago, there was a huge pot of stew—the universe. Everything was rolling around in the stew, bubbling away, and then . . . the first basic development occurred: a membrane was born.

The membrane was an amazing evolutionary leap. Without it, there was nothing to protect all the molecules in the universe from the destructive aspects of the environment. Think of this membrane as a small plastic bag. In it, molecules could develop without being attacked by the environment outside.

Over millions of years, the molecules in that primitive

Cell Division (Mitosis)

Normal Cell Division

Abnormal Cell Division
(Often found in cancer)

Centrioles
(2 pairs)   Nucleus

Centrioles
(3 pairs)   Nucleus

Chromosomes

Chromosomes

Normal – Division begins:
one pair of centrioles
duplicates.
Abnormal – Division begins:
one pair of centrioles
becomes 3 pairs.

Normal & Abnormal
Centrioles move apart.
Chromosomes appear.

Normal – Chromosomes line
up in centre plane.
Abnormal – Chromosomes
overlap in centre.

Normal & Abnormal
Chromosomes pull apart
and separate.

Normal & Abnormal
Cell begins to divide.
Nucleus re-appears.

Normal – Cell divides into
two equal cells.
Abnormal – Cell divides into
3 unequal cells.

little bag did develop, and eventually the cell as we know it today evolved. So now, we have a cell surrounded by a membrane. There are trillions of cells in one human body.

But if you were to examine one of these cells with a microscope, you'd see that in it there are even smaller bags, which are also surrounded by protective membranes. One of these bags, the most important one of all, is called the nucleus.

The nucleus of the cell contains the cell's genes, which determine such things as the color of our hair and eyes, height, and thousands of other things like that. Scientists say that the nucleus of a cell "handles its genetics."

When you start off in life, your body doesn't have trillions of cells. It has only one cell, the result of an egg uniting with a sperm. It's an amazing combination; in this first cell's nucleus are forty-six strands called chromosomes. Twenty-three are from the mother, and twenty-three are from the father.

Within each chromosome is a long line of genes which is made up of DNA, deoxyribonucleic acid.

Amazing as it seems, if you could count all the genes sitting along the chromosomes in the nucleus of one of your cells, you'd get approximately 100,000 genes. The incredible thing is, the nucleus of *every* cell in your body contains exactly the same 100,000 genes.

The second you are conceived, the egg and the sperm unite to make the first cell of the embryo. That's the blueprint—the unique set of genes that makes up a human being. Then, something happens. First, the forty-six chromosomes double. Then the nucleus of this cell divides, or splits, into two. Next the rest of the cell divides, and you end up with two cells, both exactly the same as the first cell *and* each other. Both "daughter cells," as scientists call these two new cells, have forty-six chromosomes and the same 100,000 genes. It's as if the first cell, the blueprint, went to a photocopy machine and made a couple of copies of itself. As long as the machine is working properly, those two copies will be exactly the same as the original.

Almost immediately, these two cells divide to become four

cells. Then these four cells divide to become eight cells, and then sixteen cells, and pretty soon—in nine months to be exact—you've got trillions of cells that, altogether, make up a person.

Small wonder you'd want to put a membrane around something as important as the cell's nucleus to protect its contents from all the potentially dangerous things in the environment!

I thought about Dr. Schachter's explanation for a few weeks, but there was something about it that I didn't quite follow. I understood that one cell became two cells and that two cells became four cells. And I could see that all these cells contained the same 100,000 genes. What I couldn't understand was how any one cell could possibly know that it had to become a liver cell, or a blood cell, or a brain cell.

At the very beginning, when there have been, say, only three cell divisions, there will be only eight cells, all exactly the same. They will all have the same 100,000 genes, some for hair color, others for eye color, some to produce blood, others to purify blood, and some whose sole job is to keep their cell "neat"; in fact, they are actually called housekeeping genes. But at this point, these eight cells don't produce blood, or purify blood. All they do is divide.

If the result of all this cell division is going to be a human being, rather than just a blob of dividing cells, then very soon these cells will have to differentiate—that is, become *different types* of cells such as brain cells, liver cells, blood cells, and kidney cells. How this happens, I just couldn't fathom.

How does a cell know that it's supposed to become a particular kind of cell with a specific job? How do some cells figure out that they are meant to become blood cells? And never mind just any blood cells; they have to know to become *particular kinds* of blood cells.

After all, some blood cells—the white blood cells—have the job of fighting off infection. Other blood cells—the red ones—carry oxygen around the body. Still other blood cells—the blood stem cells—have the job of reproduction;

they divide to produce new daughter blood cells as older blood cells wear out and die. These daughter blood stem cells are immature to begin with. But soon they grow into mature blood cells that are capable of performing the essential jobs taken care of by the blood in our bodies.

Another example: How do some of the first cells figure out that they have to become mature liver cells that can purify blood? Even more astounding is that mature liver cells not only know how to purify blood, they also know how to reproduce daughter liver cells. The liver is one organ that doesn't have "stem" cells whose *only* job is to reproduce daughter cells when additional cells are needed to replace those that have died. In the case of the liver, mature cells somehow know that sometimes their job is to purify blood and other times their job is to reproduce.

The first few cells of an embryo are not capable of doing any of these things. But by the time a baby is born, all the cells have figured out that they have a very special job, or jobs, to perform.

If that is going to happen, then in any particular cell, some of the 100,000 genes will have to work, and others will have to *not work*. A liver cell could not purify blood if its gene for hair production was working. A liver cell can only purify blood if its blood-purifying genes *and no other genes* (other than housekeeping genes) are in operation. What makes the whole matter even more complicated is that when it's time for the liver cell to stop purifying blood and start dividing, the genes for blood purification must stop working. And the gene for reproduction—the growth gene—must start. It's incredible that a cell could know how to do all of that.

The more I thought about it, the more impossible it all seemed. As it turned out, however, it wasn't so surprising that all this information about genes and their jobs was confusing. What seemed to me to be impossible to comprehend happens to be the tremendously complex process that baffles cancer researchers all over the world. They have been trying to understand exactly how genes work for years.

Exactly what makes some genes in a cell work and other

genes not work is one of the basic questions that scientists have spent millions of dollars trying to answer. It is also the main obstacle that keeps mankind from being able to totally understand the mystery of cancer.

How Genes Work
The remarkable question of why some genes in one cell work and other genes in the same cell do not work has to do with the process that scientists call differentiation. It means that a cell with 100,000 or so genes somehow knows that it has one, or sometimes a few, specific jobs to perform. In addition, a cell must stick to doing only one job at any one time. The job might require the activation of only a few of the cell's 100,000 genes—or sometimes, as is the case with a liver cell, different genes at different times. And it is just as important that all the other genes remain passive, or inactive.

For example, only a few out of all the 100,000 genes in a liver cell might be concerned with producing proteins that can purify blood. When that liver cell is ready to purify some blood, then the rest of its genes had better remain passive. Imagine the chaos if a gene for eye color in a liver cell suddenly started producing proteins for blue eyes, instead of proteins which are able to purify blood.

Only one of these genes in a liver cell—called the growth gene—is capable of signaling the liver cell that it's time to divide into two new cells. And it is essential that this growth gene remain inactive when the liver does not happen to need any new cells.

In the case of blood cells, this process is a bit less complicated. Any particular blood cell, unlike a liver cell, has only one job to worry about. Red blood cells carry oxygen and blood stem cells produce daughter blood cells. Therefore, a blood cell has to worry only about turning one gene on or off. When the cell is supposed to perform its one job, the appropriate gene must turn on. When the cell is not supposed to perform its job, that same gene must turn off.

But imagine for a moment what would happen if the

growth gene in a blood stem cell started working at the wrong time, that is, when the blood didn't happen to need any new blood cells. You'd get more and more and more blood stem cells. Eventually, they'd overpower the entire bloodstream.

A similar problem would occur if the growth gene in a liver cell started working at the wrong time. You'd get more and more and more liver cells. Your liver would continue to get bigger and bigger.

Turn-ons and Turn-offs
How does a gene know when it's time for it to start working or stop working? Scientists believe that mechanisms called "turn-ons" and "turn-offs" tell genes when to begin working and when to stop.

Although you'd think that most of the space on a cell's forty-six chromosomes would be taken up by all the genes, it's not so. Even more space is taken up by turn-ons and turn-offs. Unfortunately, scientists don't understand their mechanism very well. All they know is that turn-ons and turn-offs tell genes when they should start working, and when they should stop.

Take a liver cell as an example. When the body needs some blood to be purified, the environment tells the cell. Then a turn-on will signal the blood-purifying gene nearby: "Hey, the blood around here needs purifying. Produce the appropriate protein."

When some liver cells have died, perhaps of old age, the liver will get a bit too small. Again, the liver cell knows this because it is sensitive to its environment. In this case, another turn-on will say to the cell's growth gene: "I see that this liver of ours is getting a little puny. Seems we could use a few more cells." And it will signal the cell to divide.

That's what the cell's turn-ons do.

The turn-offs perform jobs that are, in some ways, even more incredible. For one thing, they make sure that all the others genes in the liver cell—the ones for hair color, eye color, height, all of which are there—don't ever turn on.

After all, it would be bedlam if a hair gene in a liver cell began to produce hair!

Once enough blood is purified, a turn-off will tell the blood-purifying gene to stop its activity, until more blood purification becomes necessary. And, after some liver cells have divided and the liver is back to the size it's supposed to be, the appropriate turn-off performs one of the body's most important jobs of all. It says "STOP!" to the growth gene. If it didn't, our livers would become disastrously large.

One of the things that happens when a person develops liver cancer is their liver becomes too big. Either the turn-off doesn't tell the growth gene to stop the reproduction process, or the growth gene no longer responds; scientists are not sure which it is. They do know that a growth gene gets turned on and for some reason, it never gets turned off again. The person who has liver cancer produces more and more and more liver cells.

To make matters worse, these liver cells aren't properly differentiated anymore. They no longer know that in addition to dividing, they are also supposed to perform another special job—purifying blood. Just like the first cells that existed when the egg and sperm had only divided a few times, these cancerous cells can't do much more than divide. They forget that they are supposed to have evolved to the point where they know not only how to divide, but how to perform other functions as well. That's another important aspect of cancer to understand: genes that are supposed to get turned on don't get turned on. Cells stop being differentiated. They cannot perform specific jobs.

Again, the mechanism for blood cells is a bit different. Normally, when the blood needs more cells, a turn-on in a blood stem cell will signal the growth gene to begin the division process and two immature daughter blood stem cells will be produced. But soon, these daughter cells mature. They differentiate into blood cells that can perform a particular job. When there doesn't happen to be a need for more blood cells, the growth gene in the blood stem cell will turn off.

When a growth gene in a blood stem cell fails to turn off, more and more blood stem cells are produced. That's one of the things that happens when a person develops leukemia, a cancer of the blood. But what makes this situation so lethal is that the daughter cells produced by a cancerous blood stem cell remain immature. They never differentiate to the point of being capable of performing a specific job. Immature white blood cells, for example, are not able to guard the body against infection.

Cancerous blood stem cells, like cancerous liver cells, are capable of only one thing—dividing. And as they divide—far more quickly, by the way, than normal cells—they compete with the rest of the body for vitamins, minerals, and other nutrients.

Cancer cells also happen to be more aggressive than normal cells. They monopolize these nutrients, becoming large enough to be called a tumor.

Eventually, a tumor can get so big that it actually presses on nearby organs, nerves, or bones. That's one of the reasons why cancer is sometimes so painful. A tumor can take over an organ completely and stop it from functioning at all. If that organ happens to be one which a person can't live without, like the liver, the person will die.

But the biggest problem is that undetected cancer tumors, and those that do not respond to treatment, can actually spread to other parts of the body. "Metastasize" is the word the doctors use. It means that a cancer cell can start off in one place and end up in another.

A cancerous liver cell, for example, can move to a lung and "seed" itself. It can grow into a cancerous liver tumor right in the lung.

Eventually, the cells from that cancerous liver might spread to a third organ and start growing a third tumor, and then to a fourth organ, and so on. Not only will the original, or primary, tumor interfere with the function of the first organ, it will also hinder the function of the organs to which it has spread.

In fact, that's the most dramatic aspect of cancer and what makes it so difficult to treat. A cancer tumor is not as difficult to deal with if it is discovered and destroyed before *even one* of its cells has had a chance to break off from the first tumor and spread.

But it is also important to understand that there is nothing about a cancer cell that is actually *poisonous*, not in the sense that a copperhead snake's venom is so deadly. Many people have the idea that cancer is like something from outer space that invades and takes over the person's body. It's not.

Cancer develops from cells that were once normal. Its deadliness comes from the fact that it spreads and, as it does, it interferes with so many of the body's normal functions that eventually nothing works at all.

Why Do Cells Become Cancerous?
It was Dr. Schachter's explanation that helped me understand what happens when someone develops cancer. Cells, for some reason we don't completely understand, lose their ability to perform properly as part of a finely balanced machine.

Why does this happen? Scientists believe that somehow, the cell's growth gene gets changed. The word they use is "mutate." Once a growth gene becomes mutated, it seems that it can also cause other mechanisms in the same cell to stop working properly, and the whole cell goes haywire. Nobody knows for sure, but many scientists believe that a cancer tumor may actually originate from one single cell that contains a mutated growth gene that has begun signaling the cell it is in to divide out of control.

Probably all the genes in all of our cells have the *potential* to change or mutate and, in fact, sometimes do.

Gene mutations are serious, but not always related to cancer. A mutation may not do any harm at all to the person in whose body it has occurred. It might, however, show up a generation or two down the road. This is the type of genetic mutation you might have read about in connection with a chemical or a drug.

Over the past few years, cancer researchers have confirmed their suspicion that specific genes are related to cancer. They now know for certain that if one of these genes becomes mutated, its cell can change into a cancer cell. So far, scientists have located twenty-two such genes, and have named them "proto oncogenes," or potential cancer genes. If and when a proto oncogene does mutate, the "proto" gets dropped and the changed gene is called an oncogene.

The name "oncogene" makes sense when you know that "onco" means "tumor," or mass. "Proto" is short for "prototype," which means "the type that occurs before." Proto oncogene is the gene that exists before a cancer gene occurs.

Research on oncogenes started in the U.S. about a decade ago. A group of scientists looked at a cancer cell, realized that it contained a mutated gene which had caused it to become cancerous, and named it an oncogene. Eventually, they realized that this oncogene had once been a perfectly normal growth gene which had somehow become mutated. That's why normal growth genes—genes that have the *potential* to mutate and cause cancer—are called proto oncogenes.

The search for something in cancer cells that could explain why they had become abnormal had taken a long time. In fact, it hadn't been possible for scientists to even begin to study genes until some amazing tiny, biochemical tools were invented. These tools could actually slice a piece of DNA into its thousands of genes so that each minuscule piece could be examined. Discovering that cancerous cells have something in common—that they contain oncogenes—was considered to be a major breakthrough in cancer research.

Proto oncogenes that have the potential to cause cancer are in the cells of every person. It's scary to think of them, like tiny time bombs ticking silently away. But most of the time they don't mutate. They remain *growth* genes and play a perfectly normal and important role in cell physiology, just like all the other genes in every cell. They control cell reproduction, turning on *if and when* cell division is required; otherwise they remain turned off.

How a Normal Gene Becomes an Oncogene

The role of these twenty-two growth genes—proto oncogenes—is to regulate cell division. Many scientists explain the theory like this: when an organ requires more cells, a turn-on signals the cell's growth gene to become active. The growth gene instructs the cell to divide. When a turn-off signals the growth gene to become inactive, the cell does not divide. As long as everything in the cell is functioning normally, a growth gene will become active only when there is a need for cell division. When there is no need, the growth gene will stay turned off; the cell will not divide; and there will be no problem.

But sometimes—a one-in-a-million chance—a growth gene will mutate into an oncogene. Just a tiny change, or more likely a couple of tiny changes, in its many parts, and it becomes an oncogene capable of changing its cell into a cancer cell.

Researchers believe that gene mutations occur most often while a cell is in the middle of dividing. Genes are most vulnerable to mutation while they are doubling.

Suppose you are in the middle of planting a new row of corn seeds in your garden right beside the row of corn seeds you planted yesterday. Let's say that the new row is the DNA of a new daughter cell, and that the seeds in this row are all its genes.

Let's also say that somehow, while you are planting this new row of corn seeds which is supposed to be exactly like the old row, you look away for a second, and someone sticks an Indian corn seed into the new row.

This is the same as if a dividing cell produced a gene for its daughter cell that wasn't quite the same as it had been in the old cell: an Indian corn seed where a regular corn seed ought to be.

That's what happens when a gene mutates. Somehow a cell that's in the middle of dividing sticks in a little piece of new cell that isn't right—a changed, or mutated, gene. Once the cell division is complete, that tiny bit of damage in the new cell will be permanent. And it will come up in all future cell divisions.

If the mutation has by chance occurred in a proto on-cogene (rather than in any other gene), changing it into an oncogene, the new cell could become a cancer cell and cause a cancerous tumor to grow. Scientists believe that more than one mutation is necessary for this to happen, and the mutations could be spaced over many years.

But say a couple of mutations do occur and a growth gene in a liver cell mutates into an oncogene. The oncogene couldn't care less whether or not the liver happens to need any more cells at that particular moment. It will turn on and signal the cell—now a cancer cell—to divide regardless. It will also cause the rest of the cell to go haywire.

Soon there will be two cancer cells, four cancer cells, then eight. Eventually, cancer cells will take over the entire liver, and it will cease to function. But exactly how all this begins is the big and still unanswered question.

So far, there are only theories about how, and why, a growth gene might mutate.

How and Why Genes Mutate

Dr. Alan Bernstein, who is working on several projects involving oncogenes for the Ontario Cancer Institute in Toronto, explained some of the theories of gene mutations.

"Scientists believe that in some instances, a growth gene, or proto oncogene, moves from the chromosome where it's supposed to be to another chromosome where it's not supposed to be. In a case like this, the mutation is in the location of the gene, rather than in the gene itself. If a proto oncogene is suddenly in the wrong place, so this theory goes, a nearby turn-on might get confused—'Who is this gene anyway, and what's it doing here?'—and signal it to turn on by mistake. This turned-on growth gene—now an oncogene—will then start signaling its cell to divide, whether new cells are needed or not. What's more, once it gets going, this oncogene will never turn off.

"In other cases, scientists believe that a proto oncogene doesn't move to another chromosome, but somehow becomes mutated right where it is. Once the gene is changed, it no longer responds properly to turn-ons and turn-offs. It just turns on and stays on, regardless of the signals it receives.

"In either case, you can imagine what will happen. The oncogene will start signaling the cell to divide, and divide, and divide."

What could cause a growth gene to move from one chromosome to another and become an oncogene? Or, what could cause a growth gene that hasn't moved to mutate into an oncogene? What is it that causes a gene that's working normally to go on the rampage?

Scientists have identified a number of things—certain chemicals, X-rays, and even a couple of viruses—that can cause human genes to mutate.

"We know that certain chemicals can cause growth genes to move or mutate," says Dr. Bernstein. "A number of the chemicals in cigarette smoke, for example, can definitely cause a growth gene to become an oncogene." Scientists have identified about thirty other chemicals in all that can cause human genes to mutate.

"In other instances," says Dr. Bernstein, "we researchers feel that the culprit is too much radiation." In laboratories, scientists have been able to demonstrate that high levels of radiation, or low levels whose effects have built up over time, can sometimes cause a gene to either move or mutate, or both.

In certain cases, scientists feel that a virus is to blame, although only two viruses have been found that can mutate human genes, and they are very rare.

"And," says Dr. Bernstein, "mutations may sometimes just happen. Maybe there's a reason and maybe it has to do with heredity; we really don't know.

"When we have been able to demonstrate that a certain substance can cause a growth gene to mutate into a cancer-causing oncogene, we call the substance a carcinogen. The word means 'cancer-causing.'"

Why Cells Follow Rules

The human body has three amazing systems that try to ensure that things don't go wrong.

The first system repairs genes that somehow get slightly damaged while they are doubling.

The second system, called the immune system, is manned by white blood cells and protects us from alien cells and microbes, such as bacteria, which sometimes invade our bodies from outside. Many scientists believe that this second system may also be able to destroy cells that have escaped the first fail-safe system and have mutated into cancer cells.

There is also a third system which ensures that cells of one type stay put in the organ where they belong. Normal liver cells can't just metastasize—that is, break off from the liver, travel to a lung, and begin living there. Cancer cells, however, can metastasize. When they grow into secondary tumors and take over a number of vital organs, they become deadly.

The first system, the one for repairing genes, works when any sort of gene becomes damaged. The damage may be caused by a carcinogen, or it may just occur spontaneously. In any case, let's suppose the damage has occurred to a gene in a cell that is right in the middle of dividing. Cells are very efficient about repairing this sort of damage. If a carcinogen does happen to cause a mutation to a gene while it is doubling, the cell can—and usually does—correct this damage.

Each cell actually has a repair shop which watches out for genetic errors. As the thousands of "bases," or tiny parts, of a new gene are being formed, this repair shop will usually notice if even one of those bases is incorrect. It also has the ability to correct a mistake *before* the dividing process is finished. When the repair shop sees a bit of new genetic material that contains an error—an Indian corn seed where a regular corn seed ought to be—it destroys this error and replaces it with the correct base.

In fact, this repair process is going on all the time. Low levels of radiation are always coming down from the sky and doing damage to genes as they double. Chemicals are frequently interfering with our lives. But the repair shop is also always on the alert, working away. It usually corrects any damage before the cell division is complete, before the damage becomes permanent and leads to more defective cells and possibly to a cancerous tumor.

But let's say that somehow—and we'll get to the reasons in Chapter 2—a gene in a dividing cell suffers some damage which the repair shop doesn't manage to catch. Suppose the repair shop misses an error, and the cell completes its division with a damaged gene—perhaps a damaged *growth* gene, an oncogene. What then? Can one of the other two systems recognize that this cell is potentially dangerous? Is one of them able to kill this abnormal cell—this cancer cell— in self-defense? In other words, is there a back-up mechanism if the first repair mechanism fails?

Some scientists believe that the answer is yes. They say that the body can get rid of at least a certain number of cancer cells that the genetic repair shop has missed. They think that the "immune system" that protects us from alien bacteria and other microbes can sometimes kill cancer cells as well.

Other researchers think that the answer is no. They say that the body probably can't get rid of cancer cells. These scientists believe that once a single cancer cell has been formed, it will, in all likelihood, go on to develop into a cancer tumor. In their opinion, the immune system can kill only alien cells, not cancer cells. While cancer cells are abnormal, they are too similar to the normal cells in a person's body to be considered alien by the immune system.

To understand these two opposing theories, it's necessary to understand a little bit about the body's immune system, which is made up of several parts. All these parts work because cells—all cells—have various types of markers that sit on their surfaces. They are called antigen markers; "I.D. cards" is how Dr. Schachter describes them.

About twenty years ago, scientists discovered one type of antigen markers called HLA markers—human leukocyte antigen markers. Ten genes on the sixth chromosome of every human cell produce ten particular proteins that move to the surface of the cell where they sit as markers and act as an amazing self-identification system.

Every cell in your body has the exact same group of ten HLA markers. Any cell that doesn't belong to your body— a bit of bacteria, a virus, even a cell from another human—will not carry these unique identifying markers. They will carry ten HLA markers, but they will be different from yours, and your body will perceive them as alien.

Around the same time, scientists also discovered that cells have hundreds of other types of antigen markers sitting on their surface.

Before they had detected these markers, scientists had known for quite a long time that our bodies have a natural defense system, the immune system, that fights against disease. But once they were able to isolate these antigen markers, they realized that the immune system has several parts and they began to figure out how each of these parts works.

One part of the immune system consists of certain white blood cells called T lymphocytes. T lymphocytes are interested in HLA markers.

A second part of the immune system consists of white blood cells called B lymphocytes. They are interested in antigen markers other than HLA markers.

A third part of the immune system consists of white blood

HLA Markers of T Lymphocyte Recognize "Self"

T lymphocyte

Body cells

HLA Markers of T Lymphocyte Distinguish "Foreign" Cell

T lymphocyte

Foreign cells

cells called NK cells—Natural Killer cells. Natural Killer cells are interested in cells that have been attacked by viruses.

T lymphocytes are produced in the lymph nodes by certain blood stem cells. At first they are immature. Then they are somehow influenced by a gland called the thymus, and they mature into T lymphocytes. In the lymph nodes of the lymphatic system—the system that keeps all the body's tissues bathed in fluid so they don't dry out—T lymphocytes are constantly on the lookout for anything that doesn't carry the ten correct HLA markers. (See illustration page 21.) You can imagine these white blood cells sidling up to every cell that passes through and comparing notes: "Are your markers the same as my markers?" If they are the same, fine. If they aren't, watch out. The T lymphocyte attaches itself to the intruder, and releases certain chemicals which kill the offending cell.

B lymphocytes are also produced by these same blood stem cells, but in the gastrointestinal tract rather than in the lymph nodes. B cell lymphocytes begin life in a very primitive form, called B cell lymphoblasts, and as they mature, they move into the lymphatic system. Eventually they mature further into plasma cells and are stored in the bone marrow.

B lymphocytes are on the lookout for anything that has foreign antigen markers on its surface. Each time the body senses the presence of a foreign antigen marker, B lymphocytes create antibodies that are designed specifically to recognize that foreign antigen marker.

These antibodies circulate through the body looking for their antigen mates. As soon as one of these antibodies spots the antigen for which it was created, it marks the cell that the antigen is on. The cell is now cited for destruction: T lymphocytes come in and finish the job.

The third part of the immune system, which is made up of NK cells, was discovered more recently than the other two parts. Scientists know much less about NK cells than about either T or B lymphocytes, but they believe that NK cells can kill cells that have been invaded by a virus.

The theory is that NK cells work in conjunction with T lymphocyte cells. While a T lymphocyte cell is busy checking out a cell's ten HLA markers, it will also notice if a foreign bit of virus is stuck to the cell's surface. If it does notice a viral antigen marker, it will signal the body to produce interferon, a chemical that can't actually kill virally infected cells, but can at least keep them from reproducing. Interferon also seems to stimulate NK cells to work harder than normal, and NK cells can kill cells that have been infected by a virus.

How Cancer Evades the Immune System
So why doesn't the immune system just kill a cell that somehow manages to mutate into a cancer cell? A cancer cell, after all, is a disease cell. If not alien, it's certainly not normal, and it can do the body terrible harm.

Scientists like Dr. Schachter don't know the answer for certain. However, some of them believe that one or more of the immune system's parts can recognize and kill a few cancer cells, at least for a while. They believe that because cancer cells divide so quickly, they soon overpower the immune system; in almost no time at all, there might be too many cancer cells for the immune system to handle. They believe that research might come up with a way of strengthening the immune system so that it can do a better job.

Other scientists believe that whatever caused the first cell to become cancerous might actually suppress the immune system, making it less able to work.

Still others believe that cancer cells themselves might produce something that prevents the immune system from working. Perhaps cancer cells can also disguise themselves in some way so that the white blood cells looking for unusual markers are fooled.

And still other scientists believe that only NK cells can kill cancer cells but, of course, NK cells would only respond to the rare types of cancer that have been caused by a virus. This is one reason why so much research has been done with interferon in recent years. Researchers have been trying to use the version of interferon that they are able to produce in labs to stimulate NK cells to work better. They have injected cancer patients with interferon and, in some cases, cancer tumors have shrunk. Unfortunately, the dream that some scientists had a few years ago—of using interferon to stimulate the immune system to fight all types of cancer—has not yielded the results that had been hoped for. It may be that interferon will work well on the rare cancers that are caused by viruses, but scientists aren't even certain about that.

"It may be," says Dr. Schachter, "that the immune system can't kill most types of cancer cells. It may be that cancer cells have the same ten HLA markers as normal cells, as well as other antigen markers for which the body produces no antibodies—because it does not consider them to be aliens." It makes sense.

"Don't forget," Dr. Schachter continues, "that a cancer cell, even though it's not functioning like a normal cell, came from a cell that was once normal. A cancer cell is not an alien, not an outsider. It's a cell from the person's own body. When you think of cancer cells that way, you can see how they might still have the right markers on their surface. While many things about a cell change when it becomes cancerous, it is possible that its markers do not change.

"It could also be that cancer cells don't have *exactly* the same markers as normal cells, but have some sort of protection on their cell surface. This protection could act as a disguise, enabling the cancer cell to trick the immune system into leaving it alone. That's another way to explain why the immune system may not kill cancer cells, why cancer cells go on dividing and dividing until eventually they form a tumor."

But that still leaves unexplained one important characteristic of cancer—metastasis. Metastasis is the most deadly aspect of this deadly disease. In an isolated organ, even if a growth gene in a cell does suffer damage and that damage escapes the first system that ordinarily repairs genes, only one cancer cell will be born. A single cancer cell is not going to hurt anybody very much.

And even if that one cancer cell does manage to escape the second control system—the immune system—and keeps dividing, only *one* cancer tumor will develop. While a cancerous tumor is extremely serious, and possibly fatal if it completely overpowers a vital organ, it would not be deadly in many, many cases *if it would only remain in the spot where it begins.*

The deadliest aspect of cancer is that it doesn't remain in one place. It spreads. Cells break off from the original tumor and metastasize to other organs, where they form new tumors. How and why cancer cells are able to do this is one of the mysteries that scientists understand least.

Says Dr. Schachter, "There must be a third marker system, one that keeps control over where a cell may live. There must be, and it must be a marker system that the cancer cell can trick."

This system must act like an airplane that takes off from a foreign airport on a scheduled flight—just a regular passenger flight, nothing suspicious. Then, after the plane takes off, it changes its route, but flies so low that it is not detected by radar. It then proceeds on a secret spy mission.

"It could be the same with a cancer cell," Dr. Schachter explains. "It could be that cancer cells trick this last failsafe system too."

First, a growth gene becomes mutated into an oncogene; the cell's first system—the repair shop—slips up, and a cancer cell is born. Next, the cancer cell tricks the second system—the immune system—into letting it alone, and the first tumor forms. Then, a cell from this tumor breaks off and tricks this third system. It makes it through radar control, so to speak, and moves to a second organ where it sets up shop. Like the airplane that flies beneath the radar detection system, the cancer cell passes all the control systems. Eventually, it "hijacks" a third organ and then moves on to a fourth. In the end, there are enough tumors to totally prohibit the body from functioning.

Some researchers, like Dr. Schachter, do believe that cancer cells probably have the same, or at least similar, markers on their surfaces as normal cells, or else some sort of protection which enables them to trick the immune system. They believe that if these markers appeared foreign, the immune system would notice a cancer cell and kill it.

But that doesn't happen. Cancer cells aren't killed; they grow. And unlike normal cells—which stick to their own kind, liver cell with liver cell, brain cell with brain cell—cancer cells can, and usually do, break off from the first tumor. These "shed" cells then move, through the bloodstream or the lymphatic system, to other parts of the body where they "seed" themselves, growing into new tumors, hijacking first one organ, then another, and eventually a third.

And the more cancer cells have spread, the harder they are to treat.

CHAPTER TWO
Who Gets Cancer?

WHO gets cancer? The terrible truth is that it will strike 30 percent—almost one in three—of the people who are living in North America today.

Cancer has been called a democratic disease. It knows no boundaries and plays no favorites; it can be found among people of all races and ages, both rich and poor, black and white, male and female. Cancer also strikes children, although it is far more common among the elderly.

One positive aspect of cancer is that it is definitely not contagious. Doctors, nurses, and researchers who treat cancer patients have no greater risk than anybody else of contracting the disease.

In fact, an unusual study was once performed on prisoners who agreed to have cancer cells transplanted from cancer patients to their own healthy bodies. These transplants never worked; the prisoners' immune systems rejected the cancer cells as "foreign." You can't get cancer by injecting cancer cells from one person into another, and you can't get cancer from being around someone—even touching or kissing someone—who has the disease.

Yet, when you know someone who has cancer, it is normal to start worrying about every bump, every pimple, every new bruise you discover on your own body. It's a terrible feeling that just about everyone has. You know in your brain that you are probably overreacting, but deep down inside, you are sure that you have cancer too. The fact is, though, you almost certainly don't.

If someone in a family has cancer, it does not become more likely that a second member of that family will develop cancer. Chances are greater, in all but a few types of cancer, that someone from another family will develop the disease. That's just the way statistics work. The odds, just like in a game of dice, tend to get spread around evenly.

Still, it's scary, there's no denying that. In North America, more than a million new cases of cancer are diagnosed every year; the disease has become more, not less, widespread in recent years.

In the 1930s, about one out of every six or seven people who lived in North America got cancer at some point during his or her life. Now it is more like one person in three.

But a closer look at the statistics reveals that the numbers are increasing, in part because medicine has made so many advances. It sounds illogical at first, but think for a minute and it will begin to make sense.

In 1930, the average lifespan was much shorter. Many people died of pneumonia, influenza, tuberculosis, diphtheria, and other diseases that medicine can now cure, or prevent by vaccination.

Prior to World War II, many young people died even before they reached adolescence. Many of them would have developed cancer if they had just lived long enough. Cancer, you see, is a disease that seems to affect people as they get older. It does strike children, but the average age of all the people in North America who are diagnosed with cancer each year is sixty-six years. Only 11,000 are under the age of twenty and only about 5,500 are under the age of ten. Almost all these young people develop leukemia, Hodgkin's disease, cancer of the brain, or the type of bone cancer, called osteogenic sarcoma, that struck U.S. Senator Edward M. Kennedy's son, Edward M. Kennedy, Jr.

Among all North Americans under the age of twenty-four, only one in 270 has had any type of cancer. The figures change, however, for people between the ages of twenty-four and fifty-five years. Of those who didn't develop cancer before the age of twenty-four, one person in seventeen will develop it before the age of fifty-five. And one person in three who makes it to the age of fifty-five will end up with some form of the disease before the age of seventy-five.

By the time you finish reading all these numbers, you may have the feeling that everyone either has cancer or is on the verge of getting it. At first, the statistics look so negative, so grim. But the truth is that most people don't get cancer. More than two-thirds of all the people you will ever meet will not develop the disease.

Of those who do get cancer, almost half won't die of it. And taking away lung cancer, which is one of the worst in terms of people actually dying, the figures look even better. Sixty percent of people who develop some type of cancer, other than lung cancer, eventually die of something else. True, that "something else" is often old age, since many people are over the age of seventy when they first develop cancer. When you look at the figures this way, they take on a different light.

Nevertheless, the big question that occupies the time of so many of today's researchers is WHO is likely to get cancer. Figures and bars and dotted lines are one thing; real people—some of whom we know and care about—are another.

Scientists called epidemiologists study groups of people who have developed a certain type of cancer and, often by a process of elimination, try to figure out what the cause of that cancer is and who else has a higher-than-average risk of developing it as well. In recent years a lot of research has related cancer to specific diets, particular chemicals, and high exposure to radiation and the ultraviolet rays of the sun.

North Americans, for example, use more fat in their diets than people of other countries in the world, and the rates of breast cancer and cancer of the colon are very high in North America. In Japan, Thailand, and India, people's diets are low in fat and these two types of cancer are comparatively rare. These findings have led epidemiologists to suggest that a high-fat diet increases a person's risk of developing breast cancer and cancer of the colon.

On the other hand, researchers have also studied the incidence of cancer in countries where people's diets are low in fat. In some of these countries—and Japan is one of them—there seems to be a relationship between diet and other types of cancer.

While there is a low rate of cancer of the colon and breast cancer in Japan, stomach cancer is relatively high. In North America, stomach cancer used to be high, but it has been declining steadily over the past thirty years and is now relatively rare. Epidemiologists believe that nutritional habits over many years may affect a person's risk of developing stomach cancer. In fact, the dietary habits people acquire during their developmental years are thought by many researchers to sometimes be the cause of a cancer that shows up two or three decades later.

In Japan, people eat a lot of foods that are preserved with nitrates and nitrites, as well as a lot of smoked foods. They also tend to eat very little of the types of fresh fruits and vegetables that contain high amounts of vitamin C. These were also the habits of North Americans until, in the 1940s, refrigeration became more accessible to the average person. Many epidemiologists believe that foods containing nitrates and nitrites contribute to stomach cancer while vitamin C actually protects people against it. They use this explanation to account for the high rate of stomach cancer in Japan and the declining rate of this disease here in North America.

But what about the two-and-a-half million people who live in a city like Chicago? Epidemiologists can compare the people of North America to the people of Japan pretty easily when they are talking about differences in diet. When they are looking at who among the people of one city are likely to get cancer, however, epidemiologists must take other factors into consideration. They can still talk about diet, for example, but the issue becomes more difficult to sort out. Other factors, such as chemicals, must be added to the discussion, and these come under the general heading of lifestyle. Some of the lifestyle factors that increase people's risk of developing cancer are ones that they themselves choose, such as smoking. Other factors, such as exposure to certain chemicals, have less to do with individual choice and more to do with environment or occupation.

Let's have another look at diet and its relationship to cancer. Both the United States and Canada are multicultural societies. Many people have immigrated to the North American continent from other countries, but nevertheless they usually stick to the dietary habits they had in their homelands.

The people who have moved to North America from Japan are a good example. It is not surprising that the people who live in the United States or Canada now, but grew up in Japan, would have a higher rate of stomach cancer than native North Americans. These people have been affected by the high-nitrate/nitrite, low–vitamin C diets they had as children in Japan. But the children of Japanese immigrants—children who were actually born in the United States or Canada, rather than Japan—also have a higher rate of stomach cancer. At first this may seem surprising, but according to most epidemiologists, the answer is still likely to be diet. Because of their cultural heritage, people carry on the dietary habits of their parents, at least for a generation or two. The third generation of Japanese North Americans, however, tends to drift away from their grandparents' type of diet toward the dietary habits of non-immigrant North Americans. And they have the same rate of stomach cancer as the rest of the North American population.

People of other cultural backgrounds also tend to develop certain types of cancer more or less frequently because of dietary habits that can change when they move. For example, many of the Eastern Europeans who migrated to North America traded their low-fat diets for the high-fat diets typical of North Americans. As they did this, their incidence of breast cancer and cancer of the colon increased.

Yet diet is only one factor. Take two people who were

born in Chicago, whose parents were born in Chicago, and who have always followed the same dietary habits. Why does one person develop cancer and not the other?

Lifestyle may be the answer. The most obvious example of a chosen lifestyle that increases the risk of developing cancer is cigarette smoking. Scientists have been able to show that, all other things being equal, a person who starts smoking cigarettes at age fifteen is thirty times more likely to develop lung cancer at age thirty-five than someone who has never smoked.

Epidemiologists have also been able to show that about thirty chemicals—vinyl chloride, which is used in the manufacture of aerosol sprays and plastics, is one example—are carcinogenic to humans. People who have worked with vinyl chloride over a period of many years are more likely to develop cancer of the liver than people who have not. Fortunately, there are now guidelines for using vinyl chloride in a way that ensures the safety of workers.

Inhaling asbestos fibers can also lead to lung cancer ten or twenty years down the road. And a smoker who works with asbestos is far more likely to develop lung cancer than a non-smoker who works with asbestos. As with vinyl chloride, guidelines have been issued for the use of asbestos, although some researchers argue that they are not tough enough.

It is true, however, that you can find two people of the same cultural heritage who live in the same city, have very similar lifestyles, and have the same type of job with the same exposure to harmful chemicals, and still one will develop cancer and the other will not.

This is a mystery that some researchers believe will someday be explained. They believe that eventually it will be possible to assess every individual and have his or her particular risk factors pinpointed. Research into genetics and immunology has been going on for approximately ten years, and already there have been some remarkable and fascinating discoveries.

Some theories suggest that a person may be more sensitive to cancer at one time in his or her life than at another time. They also suggest that some people are simply more sensitive to cancer than other people—period.

How could it really be that someone might be more sensitive to cancer at one time in his or her life than at another? One explanation has to do with age: As people get older, they may become more susceptible to cancer. Another explanation has to do with cell division. If a person's cells begin to divide more frequently than usual—and that can happen at any age for any number of reasons—then the simple law of averages says that the genes in those cells have more chances of becoming mutated. This is especially true if the cells are being bombarded by a carcinogen during the period of rapid division.

Consider the aging theory. By the time people are elderly, they have had many opportunities to be exposed to carcinogens. Also, the mechanisms in an old body begin to wear out. Eighty-year-old knees don't bend as well as they did at age twenty-five. By the same token, researchers suggest that surveillance systems might also begin to wear out as people age. The repair shop that watches out for genetic errors during cell division might not be as efficient as it once was. The immune system may wear down and not recognize antigen markers quite as well; NK cells may not respond to interferon, or perhaps less interferon is produced. Perhaps the system which prevents cells from metastasizing doesn't work quite as well either.

Scientists don't have the answers for these questions. They do know that the average age of cancer patients is sixty-six, and from this, they theorize that older people are probably more susceptible to cancer than people who are young.

It is frightening to think that during some periods of life a person may be more sensitive to a carcinogen than during other periods. But if you think about how and when cells divide, this too will begin to make sense.

Remember the example of an Indian corn seed being planted by mistake in a row of regular corn seeds? When a cell is dividing, it is more sensitive to a carcinogen than when it is not dividing. It follows, then, that if cells in a particular organ start dividing rapidly—far more rapidly than is normal—there will be more chances for a genetic error to be made. The more errors that are made, the harder it would be for the genetic repair shop to keep up.

Imagine a table fan on a desk on a hot summer day. If the fan is turned off and its blades are just turning a little in the breeze, you could throw a wrench into the fan and do very little damage. But turn the fan on high speed, and then throw in a wrench. The blades would look like spaghetti in a second.

The interesting question is why your cells would be dividing more quickly at one time in your life than at another. Why would they ever be dividing so quickly that the repair shop couldn't keep up?

If a lot of cells suddenly die for one reason or another, then a lot of rapid cell division would be necessary to replace them. Normally cell division occurs relatively slowly. A cell dies. It is replaced. Another one dies; it is replaced.

It is true that some cells, such as blood cells, multiply very rapidly compared with the other cells, such as liver cells. But as far as the blood cells' reproduction system is concerned, their normal rate of division is not too fast for the genetic repair shop to keep up. This system is meant to work quickly, and few errors escape inspection.

Other systems are not designed to work as quickly. One instance when cells could be dividing too quickly for the repair shop to keep up is when skin becomes sunburned.

If you sunbathe without using a sunscreen, your skin will burn, and the body must make new skin cells. Millions of skin cells die all at once and they must be replaced very quickly. There is, therefore, an abnormally high amount of cell division going on, which makes it difficult for the genetic repair shop to keep up with any errors that might occur. And to make matters worse, while this quick division is going on, more carcinogenic ultraviolet rays are hitting the skin cells.

Another example is a person with a lung infection such as bronchitis. When someone has bronchitis, the lungs become inflamed, meaning that many lung cells have died.

To replace those that have been lost, lung cells begin dividing quickly. Again, it is difficult for the lung's genetic repair shop to keep up.

Now imagine that while this rapid cell division is occurring, a person is also smoking. The chances that the carcinogens in the cigarette smoke will damage a gene in a lung cell are far greater while the lung cells are dividing rapidly. The law of averages also says that the chances are greater that the affected gene will be a growth gene. If it is, a cancer cell will be born.

The other theory suggests that some people might simply be more sensitive to cancer-causing substances than other people—not just on certain occasions, but all the time.

The most obvious explanation for this is that one person's genetic repair system might not work as well as another person's, regardless of age and lifestyle.

After all, John McEnroe is a better tennis player and Mikhail Baryshnikov is a better dancer than most people—no matter how hard those other people try. Maybe one person's T and B lymphocyte cells are just better at recognizing subtle differences in HLA and other antigen markers than another person's.

Although scientists don't know for sure, some believe that even the system that prevents metastasis may work better in one person's body than in another person's, even though they are the same age. That would explain why similar cancer tumors sometimes spread, or metastasize, more quickly in one person than in another.

All these theories are being investigated by researchers, and already some interesting experiments have taken place.

People with red hair and light skin tend to get skin cancer more often than people with brown hair and darker skin. Why? Probably because the red-haired person's skin burns more easily. Light skin contains less of the substance called melanin, which protects skin cells from the ultraviolet rays of the sun and from carcinogenic chemicals in the environment.

Since red-haired, light-skinned people burn more easily,

their skin cells would be damaged sooner than dark-haired, darker-skinned people's skin cells. Because redheads' skin cells are dividing rapidly for longer, there are simply more opportunities for damage to take place.

Some explanations are more complex than the amount of melanin in someone's skin. Lung cancer has been directly linked to cigarette smoking. Of the more than 150,000 North Americans who develop lung cancer each year, few are non-smokers. But why is it that many smokers do not develop lung cancer? Why one person, but not another?

An explanation by Dr. Zsolt Harsanyi, an American scientist who, with writer Richard Hutton, co-authored the book *Genetic Prophecy: Beyond the Double Helix,* suggests that there might be something about one person's lung cells that makes him or her more susceptible to lung cancer than another person.

According to Dr. Harsanyi, when you inhale smoke from a cigarette, a bunch of different chemicals enter your lungs. Some of these chemicals are perfectly harmless. The lungs dissolve them and they are carried to the kidneys by the bloodstream. In the kidneys, they are processed further and then they are excreted as waste.

But other chemicals in cigarette smoke are not as easily dissolved. What's worse, they are actually poisonous. Some, like tars, also become carcinogenic when they are chemically altered even slightly.

The lungs will not tolerate poisons that could eventually build up to what are called "toxic" levels, which could cause death. In their desire to cleanse themselves, they try to get rid of these poisons. Certain genes in certain lung cells produce specific proteins, called enzymes, which turn these poisons into substances that can be dissolved in the bloodstream. Once in the bloodstream, they can travel to the kidneys to be disposed of once and for all.

One particular group of undissolvable poisons in cigarette smoke are tars called polycyclic hydrocarbons. These tars can become carcinogens with only a minor chemical change.

A special group of enzymes, produced by a special group

of genes, works on these hydrocarbons to get them into a form that can be dissolved in the bloodstream.

Dr. Harsanyi describes these enzymes as if they were workers in a factory assembly line. Each gene, or factory worker, produces an enzyme that either adds to, or chops off, a different part of a hydrocarbon. With each step, the hydrocarbon gets a little closer to a dissolvable form.

Now it happens that one of these enzymes—one that works somewhere in the middle of the chain—is called AHH, which stands for aryl hydrocarbon hydroxylase. The problem with AHH is that while it does make a hydrocarbon more dissolvable, it also changes it into a carcinogen.

Normally, if the body is working well and all the factory worker genes are in tune with one another, this cancer-causing stage doesn't last very long. The next factory worker in the line comes along and converts the hydrocarbon still further—into a substance that is no longer cancer-causing.

But suppose the gene in the assembly line that produces the AHH enzyme is overactive. If that happens, then the next gene in the chain won't be able to keep up. The hydrocarbon will get to the cancer-causing stage in the chain and remain there for a relatively long period of time.

The more cancer-causing substances that are produced, and the longer they remain in the lungs, the more likely it is that they will cause genetic damage. If they happen to cause a growth gene to mutate into an oncogene, a cancer cell will be born.

But just as scientists ask why some people have light skin that produces low amounts of melanin, they ask why other people have a gene that produces too much AHH.

They ask, but at the moment they can't answer. It's like asking why some people are tall and others are short. It has to do with heredity. Why one child will inherit one particular trait, and another child in the same family will not, is another of the amazing mysteries of life—and, perhaps, the luck of the draw.

It's easy to see who has light skin and is therefore more sensitive to skin cancer, but finding a gene that produces too much AHH is tricky and very expensive. There are very few genetic research centers with the gene-slicing equipment necessary to begin studying genes. Even fewer of these laboratories are dedicated to cancer research. It's not possible for a family doctor doing a check-up to analyze genes. And it's unlikely that this situation will change in the near future.

Still, some scientists hope that if enough money is put into this type of genetic research, significant progress will be made.

Scientists may someday develop a simple, inexpensive way to determine whether one person is more sensitive to the poisons in cigarette smoke than another person because of basic genetic differences. For all smokers, the chances of developing lung cancer are one in ten. But imagine if scientists could narrow the risk for certain people to one in three, or one in two. Imagine if they could tell a person, "Look, if *you* smoke, given your genetic makeup, it will be amazing if you *don't* develop lung cancer." Imagine that!

At the moment, it can't be done, not with lung cancer anyway. But scientists are starting to identify other genes that seem to point to certain types of cancer.

Scientists have learned that retinoblastoma, a rare form of eye cancer that affects children under the age of four, is one of the few types of cancer that tends to occur in the brothers and sisters of children who have this disease. They also know that retinoblastoma is due to a genetic abnormality—the absence of a number of genes on the thirteenth chromosome. Doctors will therefore keep the brothers and sisters of retinoblastoma patients under strict surveillance and will usually be able to detect the disease at an early stage, when it can be cured without the child having to lose an eye. Looking for answers to medical questions through genetics is starting to become more and more common.

Researchers are also beginning to link genetic abnormalities to other, more common types of cancer. Breast cancer and cancer of the kidney are among the ones that are now being investigated.

Our hope for the future in this type of research is almost

limitless. It might mean that some day doctors could warn a person to watch out for a certain type of cancer, or a certain cancer-causing chemical, to which he or she might be particularly vulnerable. Not only would our society have a general knowledge about things that increase the risk of cancer, but each person would have his or her own special risk-factor scheme.

What we are talking about, of course, is prevention: the idea that the best cure for cancer may be making sure that people don't get it at all.

CHAPTER THREE
Prevention

I N 1960, President John F. Kennedy announced that there would be a person on the moon before the end of the decade. Incredible as it seemed at the time, Kennedy was making a safe bet. He knew it was possible. Succeeding was only a matter of hard work and money.

The rockets existed; they just weren't powerful enough. The materials for space suits existed; they just weren't tough enough. What was needed were some adjustments to what already existed rather than something completely new. By 1960, a craft had already been put into space. Getting one onto the moon, with an astronaut in it, was a matter of improving something scientists already knew how to do. It happened, of course, in the summer of 1969.

Finding the ultimate cure for cancer, however, is not like getting astronaut Neil Armstrong onto the moon. Another president, Richard M. Nixon, found that out after he announced, in 1972, that Americans would find a way to eradicate cancer from the face of the earth by the beginning of the 1980s.

The fact that President Nixon's dream still hasn't been realized is nobody's fault. Finding the ultimate cure to cancer is a lot tougher to achieve than putting a person onto the moon. As Dr. Schachter explained, finding that cure involves understanding the cause or causes of cancer at a cellular level, and that involves learning the answers to some basic cellular principles about which scientists are just beginning to gain some understanding.

And yet, in spite of all the depressing figures about the number of deaths from cancer each year, a lot is happening in the field of cancer research that is positive. One of the most positive developments is in the area of prevention—preventing cancer through an examination of our environment. The word "environment" is meant to include diet, as well as chemicals, radiation, and viruses.

Right now, with the knowledge scientists already have, cancer can frequently be prevented. In fact, some researchers believe that cancer is preventable as much as 80 or 90 percent of the time. These researchers believe that although we don't know the basics of how cancer begins, we do know many of its environmental causes, most of which are within our control.

Dr. Anthony Miller, director of epidemiology for the National Cancer Institute of Canada, has broken the causes of cancer into four groups. Diet, he believes, accounts for between 35 and 50 percent of all cancers. He emphasizes, however, that this field is complex, and that researchers have not yet sorted out all the relationships between cancer and food.

Chemicals, Dr. Miller believes, account for approximately 40 percent of all cancers, but only about 5 percent of those are chemicals other than cigarette smoke. Radiation and viruses, he says, account for another 3 or 4 percent of all cancers. If you add all these percentages, you get approximately 93 percent; only 7 percent of cancers remain unaccounted for.

When faced with statistics such as these, many people agree with Dr. Miller that prevention is the most important area of cancer research. They believe that as much money should be spent on prevention—learning more about the exact environmental causes of cancer and educating more people to consider them—as is spent on other types of research and treatment. At the moment, relatively little of the money raised by the American and Canadian Cancer Societies is earmarked for prevention. Nevertheless, while "basic" researchers and "applied" researchers continue to work on basic answers, and on ways of applying these answers to patients, epidemiological researchers like Dr. Miller continue their work in the area of prevention. Each year they uncover more and more answers to cancer's environmental links.

The concept of cancer prevention began two hundred years ago, when Dr. Percival Pott noticed that many of his scrotal cancer patients had worked as chimney sweeps when they were young boys—far too many for it to be merely coincidental. Although the science, or even the word "epidemiology," had not yet been invented, Dr. Pott was the world's first epidemiologist.

It seemed like a good idea to consider why so many chimney sweeps were developing cancer of the scrotum, and so Dr. Pott began asking his patients for details of their lives. Many told him that as children, sweeping chimneys, they had rarely washed or changed their soot-stained clothes. They said they had been too poor to afford more than one set of clothing, and bathtubs were not exactly the norm in the 1700s. Dr. Pott theorized that over the years the powerful carcinogens in the burned coal had been absorbed into the chimney sweeps' skin. These carcinogens, he believed, had caused scrotal cancer to appear decades later.

While Dr. Pott was astute enough to look at the statistics and realize that something in soot must be causing the scrotal cancer, the Danes were the first people to practice cancer prevention as a nation. They passed a law stating that all chimney sweeps had to wash and change their soot-stained clothes each day after work. When the number of cases of scrotal cancer began to decline in Denmark, other nations began to follow suit.

It was not, however, for almost two hundred years that the most important discovery in cancer prevention was made. In the early 1950s, the first articles linking cigarettes to the most deadly cancer of all, lung cancer, appeared in American and British scientific journals. Over the next few years, more articles appeared. Then, in 1962, the British Royal College of Physicians published a report on smoking and health. In 1964, U.S. Surgeon General Dr. Luther Terry did the same. Both reports stated that the chance of developing lung cancer increases with the number of cigarettes a person smokes.

Dr. David Nostbakken is president of the International Liaison Committee for Smoking and Health. "Up until 1964," he says, "the smoking public puffed away, unaware of the health hazard. There was, I suppose, a general feeling that smoking wasn't exactly *good* for you. But the real evidence that conclusively links cigarettes to cancer was not known when my parents were teenagers. Many people have lung cancer today because they became addicted to cigarettes during the years when we were still so naive. Now that we do know, however, we could eventually prevent a third of all cancer deaths . . . if we could only convince young people not to start smoking."

You'd think that it would be easy to convince teenagers not to smoke. Studies show that a teenager who begins smoking a pack a day at age fifteen is thirty times more likely to develop lung cancer by age thirty-five than one who has never smoked. And yet studies also indicate that the age at which teenagers are starting to smoke has actually gone down, from fifteen years to twelve years.

How can this be? People like Dr. Nostbakken blame the tobacco companies, with their multimillion-dollar advertising campaigns; in North America, the tobacco industry spends close to three billion dollars a year— $3,000,000,000—trying to promote smoking as both sophisticated and healthy. According to Dr. Nostbakken, young people fall for these ads.

The tobacco companies insist that they are not interested in trying to convince young people to smoke. They claim that the purpose of their advertising is merely to get smokers to change brands—as if even *that* would be ethical. Meanwhile, each time I look at another new ad which pictures smoking hand in hand with sophistication—and even sports—I become more and more skeptical about trusting these claims.

In 1984, when tobacco manufacturer RJR-Macdonald Inc.

began to sponsor the Canadian Ski Association with the "Export A Cup," there was no longer any doubt in my mind. If tobacco companies are not really interested in getting young people to smoke, why are they so keen to spend millions of dollars sponsoring amateur ski events where the majority of participants and fans are under the age of eighteen? Why do their ads suggest that young people who live the good life always smoke? And why do they have representatives at sports stadiums handing out free packages of cigarettes to kids?

The answer is simple. Tobacco companies are not in business to lose money, but to sell tobacco to whomever they can convince to buy it, and they couldn't care less if that person is sixteen or eighty-six years old.

Dispelling the sophisticated image of smoking is tackled by the American and Canadian Cancer Societies and a few other organizations. Unfortunately, they have relatively few dollars to spend. Until there is more money for this purpose, Americans and Canadians will probably continue to spend more than twenty-five billion dollars a year on cigarettes, and more than twenty billion dollars on health care costs because of cigarettes. More than 150,000 North Americans a year will continue to develop lung cancer. And, because lung cancer is almost always impossible to treat successfully, close to the same number will die. It's a bittersweet notion that we know how to prevent lung cancer, but don't.

Skin cancer is another type of cancer we know how to prevent, but don't. In North America, almost 500,000 new cases of skin cancer are diagnosed every year, mostly because of overexposure to the ultraviolet rays of the sun without the protection of a sunscreen.

Many people overexpose themselves to sunshine because of tough-to-resist advertising. In this case, the ads try to make us believe that suntans are beautiful and, ironically enough, healthy.

It is lucky that skin cancer is not the killer that lung cancer is. Almost all the 500,000 people who develop skin cancer each year can be cured.

In other cases, however, people have applied the knowledge about prevention that epidemiologists have uncovered. For example, luminous watch paint that glows in the dark contains radium and has been linked to bone cancer. Sixty years ago, factory workers used this type of paint to draw numbers on watches. They dipped their brushes into the paint and, to get a fine point, tipped them against their tongues.

Obviously, these workers were swallowing a certain amount of the paint and, although no one was aware of it, the radium in it was settling in their bones. When many of these workers developed bone cancer, the connection was eventually made, the practice stopped, and the incidence of bone cancer declined.

Over the years, scientists have learned other things about the relationship between radiation and cancer. Twenty-five years ago, for example, children who were being fitted for shoes had their feet exposed to radiation by machines that used X-rays to show how the shoes fit. I can remember giggling at the picture of my own toes squiggling inside a "magic" machine. These machines have long since been banned.

From the late 1930s until the mid-1940s, some North American children whose thymus glands were found to be abnormally large were treated with radiation. This reduced the size of the gland. This treatment has since been discontinued. It is essential, however, that anyone who had this treatment during childhood consult a physician who can determine if there have been any adverse effects from the radiation. The treatment is thought to have increased the risk of tumor in the thyroid gland, which is positioned in front of the thymus.

Since Dr. Percival Pott identified soot as a carcinogen, about thirty additional chemicals have been shown to cause cancer in humans. Many of them are now avoided. You may remember when newspaper articles about the cancer-causing properties of asbestos started to appear. Before the early 1970s, asbestos was commonly used as a building material because it was both fireproof and an excellent insulator. When scientists realized that asbestos is also a powerful carcinogen, its use was reduced.

Other chemicals that we now avoid—or at least use carefully—include vinyl chloride, the cleaning fluid carbon tetrachloride, and a type of solvent called benzene.

Identifying carcinogenic chemicals is only one of the many areas of cancer prevention. Scientists have also developed tests which can detect cancer in its earliest stages. In these cases, they are not able to prevent cancer completely, but they are able to prevent it from becoming a life-threatening disease.

Most of the time, for instance, death from cervical cancer can be prevented because it can be detected at a very early stage. This is due to the work of a Greek physician, George Papanicoulaou, who invented the Pap test, a simple, painless procedure that takes less than a minute for a physician to perform.

A swab of cells from the cervix—it's as easy as scraping a few cells from the inside of the cheek—are smeared onto a piece of glass and then studied in the lab. From the way the cells look, cancer can be detected and cured completely *before* it progresses. It's an amazing preventive technique that has saved the lives of thousands of women all over the world.

Scientists have also learned, for example, that people who develop polyps—tiny growths in the colon—have a higher-than-average risk of developing cancer of the colon *if* these non-cancerous polyps are not treated. Now a careful watch is kept on these patients and the polyps are removed before the cancerous changes have had a chance to take place. Many physicians have praised President Ronald Reagan's decision to be open and honest about his own experience with cancer of the colon. It is hoped that, as a result, many other high-risk people will become more diligent about ensuring that they have frequent examinations.

Progress is being made in the detection of breast cancer as well. There are now several ways of detecting breast cancer at an early stage, the easiest being breast self-examination—BSE. Studies have shown that women who know how to do BSE properly can detect early breast tumors that are no larger than a pea. On the other hand, breast tumors discovered by accident have often grown to the size of a golf ball. Death from breast cancer can be prevented 85 percent of the time if it is detected at an early stage. Today, more and more women are being diagnosed with breast cancer at this early stage.

Very little is heard about stomach cancer anymore. In Chapter 2, I mentioned that the decline in the incidence of this disease has to do with the decline in the use of such preservatives as nitrates and nitrites, and the increase in the use of fresh fruit and vegetables, particularly those that are high in vitamin C. Epidemiologists are responsible for our knowledge of nitrates, nitrites, and vitamin C. In North America, in the 1930s, approximately thirty-four new cases of stomach cancer were reported each year for every 100,000 people. By 1980 there were only about eight cases per 100,000 people.

Recently, researchers have come up with even more information that links certain types of cancer to certain types of food. What remains to be seen is whether or not we will use this knowledge. It will mean changing our dietary habits—the lifestyle we have become accustomed to over the past thirty or forty years.

A high-fat diet increases a person's risk of developing cancer of the colon and the rectum, cancer of the prostate in men, and breast cancer in women. Both the American and Canadian Cancer Societies, which have always been cautious about linking diet to cancer, are now suggesting that the average North American can reduce his or her risk of developing cancer by dietary changes.

They are advising us to eat less fat: no more than 30 percent of the calories consumed daily should be made up of fat. This means cutting down on fatty meats and whole milk products: cream, ice cream, and high-fat yogurt. An interesting study on animals that is in no way conclusive for humans suggests that the fat contained in meats may have a more adverse affect than the fat contained in milk products. More studies in this area are being conducted.

To cut down on their fat intake, people must replace high-fat products with other foods. High-fiber-content foods such as fruit, vegetables, and whole grains are recommended. These may even decrease a person's risk of developing cancer, although scientists' opinions on this issue are still divided.

A diet rich in vitamins C and A is thought to decrease the risk of developing certain types of cancer.

Vitamin C is thought to protect humans against stomach cancer and cancer of the esophagus, probably because it neutralizes the effects of preservatives such as nitrates and nitrites. In fact, many of the foods preserved with nitrates and nitrites now contain vitamin C as well.

The information so far on vitamin A, which is also called carotene, is sketchier. Studies done on animals, and a few on humans, suggest that vitamin A may lower the risk of cancer of the larynx, esophagus, and lung. Carrots contain vitamin A, as do apricots, cantaloupes, tomatoes, spinach, and peaches.

Scientists point out, however, that popping vitamin A supplements is not a good idea, since excessive amounts of this vitamin can be toxic. I went to school with a boy who, after six weeks of eating nothing but carrots and vitamin A supplements, turned an amazing shade of orange. As they carted him home from the hospital after tests, the doctor said he had overdosed on carotene!

Dr. Miller also points out that while spinach contains vitamin C, it also contains nitrates. Young people who are interested in getting out of eating spinach might want to note this epidemiological point.

Some research has suggested that "brassica" type vegetables, such as cabbage, broccoli, brussels sprouts, cauliflower, and kohlrabi, may reduce the risk of cancer of the colon and cancer of the rectum. That's because brassica vegetables contain certain impossible-to-pronounce chemicals such as isothiocynates, indoles, flavones, and phenols.

Heavy drinkers of alcohol, especially those who also smoke, have an unusually high risk of developing oral cancer as well as a disease of the liver called cirrhosis, which sometimes leads to liver cancer. Researchers believe that something in the distillation process of alcohol causes it to become carcinogenic to a minor degree. Both the American and Canadian Cancer Societies recommend that people be moderate in their consumption of alcohol.

Moderation is also the word where smoked and salt-cured foods, as well as nitrates and nitrites, are concerned. The amount of nitrate and nitrite that can, by law, be used as a preservative was reduced some years ago. Hams, fish, and some types of sausage, which are smoked in the traditional way, absorb cancer-causing tars during the smoking process. These tars are similar to the ones found in cigarette smoke. There is also some evidence that links salt-cured or pickled food to cancer of the stomach and esophagus.

Can we change our diets? The recommendations to eat more fruits and vegetables that contain vitamin C and vitamin A, whole grains, and fewer processed foods, should be fairly easy habits to assimilate. The recommendation to drink alcohol only in moderation will probably be the same as it has always been—easy for some people, difficult for others.

Reducing the amount of fat in our diets could cause problems. Already there have been some noises from certain industries which, like the tobacco industry, have a great deal at stake. The dairy industry, for example, could transfer some of its profits from whole milk and high-fat yogurt to skim milk, and to low-fat yogurt. But what about ice cream? And what about the beef industry? On certain cuts of beef, it is difficult to trim fat away. Some researchers are worried that the beef industry, which doesn't make huge profits to begin with, may not feel like taking this latest health edict lying down.

In the end, will we, as a society, change our eating habits? Or will a political battle similar to the one launched by the tobacco companies emerge? It's hard to say; beef-eaters and milkshake-lovers don't pollute the environment in the same way smokers do. It is doubtful that the proponents of low-fat diets will launch a campaign that has the ferocity of the non-smokers' rights organizations.

In any case, the answer to whether or not 35 to 50 percent of cancer will someday be prevented through dietary changes is not in the hands of adults. This question will be answered in the future by teenagers who must decide if they want to make new choices. In the future, epidemiologists will likely discover even more about cancer prevention. Like the science of genetics, the study of cancer and diet is a relatively new field. As well, thousands of new chemicals are developed each year and each must be tested to determine if it has carcinogenic properties.

One thing, however, is clear. Prevention, like basic research, is an exciting field. If we already have the knowledge to prevent approximately 80 percent of all cancer, who would want to argue that going further in the area of epidemiology and education is less important than discovering a cellular cure?

CHAPTER FOUR
Treatment—Living with Cancer

LEARNING about prevention is exciting for people who don't have cancer, or who don't know someone who does. Learning about genes, and what a deeper knowledge of their function will mean someday in terms of eradicating cancer, is exciting too. But today, this very year, more than a million North Americans have found out that they have cancer. What is happening to them?

Most of them are being treated by one of the several thousand oncologists who work in American and Canadian hospitals. Oncologists are physicians who specialize in cancer treatment. The "onco" part of the word comes from the same Greek word as the "onco" in oncogene: *onkos* means "tumor," or mass.

Dr. Richard Hasselback is one of these oncologists. He treats cancer patients at the Princess Margaret Hospital in Toronto, where he has been working for twenty-three years. He is well aware of the truth—that treatment will be successful for fewer than half of the people who become cancer patients this year.

But Dr. Hasselback has also seen some exciting advances over the years. And he knows that five years from now—five is the number of years it takes until most types of cancer are considered "cured"—almost half of these people will join the ranks of the three-and-a-half million people living in North America today who have fought cancer and won.

Matthew is one of these people. Six years ago, a doctor extracted a blood sample from a vein in Matthew's left arm, sent it to a lab, and got back a report that indicated an abnormal number of white blood cells. The next day, Matthew was hospitalized for a "bone marrow aspiration" test to determine if his blood-producing cells—his blood stem cells—were cancerous. They were. The diagnosis was acute leukemia, cancer of the white cells of the blood. At the time, Matthew was thirty-eight years old. He was married to Diana, and they had three children. Aubrey was fourteen; Lillian was eight; and little Sol was only three.

Matthew: "It happened just before Christmas. There was no snow that year." Even now it takes Matthew a few moments to build up to talking about his experience with cancer. "I had been exhausted for weeks. I didn't want Diana to worry, so I went to see Jack, our family doctor, on my own. Hell, it was probably nothing more than a lingering, low-grade infection. But I think now, in my heart, I must have known."

The next two days were a tornado. Matthew had the blood test and then the bone marrow aspiration. An oncologist was called in for consultation and his treatment with chemicals—chemotherapy, they call it—was started the same night.

Certain things about the three most frequently used treatments for cancer have changed over the years. But in many ways, they are the same basic treatments that physicians like Dr. Hasselback had to choose from twenty years ago: surgery, radiation therapy, and chemotherapy (which is used far more often today than in the past).

Matthew: "Treatment! I didn't think about treatment. I don't think it even crossed my mind that my chances were less than fifty-fifty, that the drugs they were pumping into my vein were the only thing between me and death. All I could think about was Diana and the kids. How in the world was this going to affect them?"

Diana: "I was numb. Swirling around in my brain were a thousand thoughts. I couldn't imagine how I was going to cope. A part of me was asking, 'Why *me*?' Just when Sol is getting old enough to go to nursery school. Just when

I can finally have a bit of time for myself again, go back to work, feel a bit free. I've talked to other women in my position. Everyone is different, of course, but many have said much the same thing. There is such a jumble of feelings. I felt devastated. I felt nauseous. Angry. Depressed. Overwhelmed and sorry for myself, all at the same time. Looking back, I think I also felt guilty for not being able to be totally sensitive to what Matthew must have been going through—for thinking of myself when he was the one who might die. I wish I had known then that just about everyone has to cope with these conflicting emotions."

Aubrey, the oldest, remembers the night when Matthew was hooked up to the intravenous tube, the I.V., that would deliver those drugs: "I'd never seen him like that before. He was so . . . twitchy. I can't think of any other word. I was there, you know, for half an hour, and he kept going on about the weather and my school. It was crazy. Mom had said he had something really important to tell us. I mean, you don't exactly go into the hospital for the good of your health!" Aubrey pauses for a few seconds for emphasis. He looks pleased with himself for making the little joke. Six years ago, however, joking around was a little harder.

Matthew: "Kids have this idea about their parents. Hell, I'm forty-four now and I still have the same fantasy about my own mother and father. You think that because parents are adults, they can handle these crises without cracking up. I'm a pretty open guy. I believe in sharing my feelings with my family. But I can tell you, I felt about six years old the night I had to tell my kids.

"I remember hearing myself blurt it out after what seemed like hours of talking about nothing. Saying the word 'cancer' was the hardest part of all. After that, telling them that it was leukemia, and that I might die, didn't seem very difficult."

Aubrey: "Yup, so that was it. He finally worked up to saying it: cancer. What did I know about cancer? But, you know, when he said it, suddenly I figured it would be okay. I think now, looking back, it was that he trusted us enough to say it. I never thought he would die."

When you start to talk about whether a person with cancer will live or die—and it is a horrible thing to think of someone you love as part of a winning or losing group—you have to talk about many, many things. One of them, of course, is which type of cancer that person has.

Almost no one with skin cancer or lip cancer, for example, dies of their disease. These are not the most serious kinds of cancer in the sense that they are almost always discovered early, treated, and cured.

At the other end are lung cancer, liver cancer, and cancer of the pancreas. Very few of the people with one of these types of cancer make it to the end of those critical first five years. The reasons are complicated. But basically, cancers like these are so hard to cure because they are asymptomatic in their early stages; that is, there are no signs or symptoms. Because of this, they are rarely discovered before they have advanced too far to be treated successfully.

Most of the other types of cancer are in the middle of these two extremes. Breast cancer, some types of leukemia, cancers of the lymphatic system, cancers of the bone, the uterus, the rectum, and the colon are all in a huge gray area. When a person is diagnosed with one of these kinds of cancer, the outcome can almost always go either way. Living in this gray area, sometimes for years, can be one of the most difficult aspects of cancer with which people must cope.

But another even more stressful aspect of cancer treatment is a general statement that cancer patients, or their families, often hear: that the *overall success rate* for treatment has not changed all that much over the past thirty years.

Is the statement true? "Yes and no," is how Dr. Hasselback explains it: "It's true, but the main reason why the overall figures for cancer treatment have not changed over the past thirty years has to do with lung cancer.

"The death rate for cancer of the colon is down—although only slightly.

"Breast cancer has stayed the same, but you can say that

we are doing better with the *treatment* of breast cancer today in one sense. More women are developing breast cancer today than in the past. Nevertheless, only about the same number of women are dying of it each year. This means that the treatment is successful in more cases.

"Deaths from certain types of leukemia, Hodgkin's disease, testicular cancer, thyroid cancer, stomach cancer, and cancer of the cervix have declined dramatically. Successes have come because of treatment for the first four, because of prevention in the case of stomach cancer, and because of early discovery in the case of cancer of the cervix.

"But lung cancer . . ." Dr. Hasselback's voice remains steady, but it's not difficult to get a sense of how he feels. "If it weren't for the fact that the number of people who develop lung cancer and die from it continues to go up, the overall cure rate for cancer would be improving, not staying the same."

Dr. Miller confirms what Dr. Hasselback has to say. "If lung cancer were wiped out—that is, if cigarettes were suddenly obliterated from the face of the earth—the number of deaths from lung cancer would all but stop, and deaths from cancer in general would eventually decline by a third."

The picture is fairly black and white when you talk about the easy-to-treat cancers on the one hand, and the almost-impossible-to-treat varieties on the other. But the discussion of survival and death is a much more complex matter for most other types of cancer.

Often, when cancer is first detected, it is impossible for the doctors to say for certain if a particular person will live or die.

Matthew: "How can I even begin to describe what I thought about life and death during those first few weeks? Would the anti-cancer chemicals they were shooting into me kill my cancer cells, or would my cancer cells kill me? One minute I was sure I'd live. The next minute I'd figure I'd had it. . . . I tried so hard not to take out the anger and self-pity I felt about being in this position on Diana and the kids. But I know there were many times when I failed. They all tell me now that I mostly said I was sorry when I jumped on them for nothing. But sometimes I wonder if they just say it to make me feel a little better."

Aubrey: "It's true. A lot of the time during that first month he was a yo-yo—up one day, down the next. I think we all were. One day I'd understand why he was in a bad mood and sympathize. I knew the drugs were making him sick as a dog and that he was scared half to death. But the next day I'd think, 'Do I need this? Here I am giving up my weekends to sit here with him. The least he can do is appreciate me.' "

Matthew: "But try to see it from where I was at—the panic, the incredible stress that stays with you twenty-four hours a day. You're living with it. It's inside of you, so you can make some sense out of it. I've talked to other cancer patients and we all seem to ask ourselves the same thing: is it possible to explain all this to kids who have lives of their own and less experience with stress? I thought if I told them I was terrified that I'd die, it would scare them. On the other hand, if I kept everything to myself, I ran the risk of having them think I was angry at *them*."

Diana: "Some days I'd go to the hospital and Matthew wouldn't want to talk. Other days, you couldn't shut him up! I tried to let him take the lead as much as I could. The hardest part for me was talking about our finances. I wanted him to be totally positive, perhaps unrealistically so. But I knew in my heart that he needed to know that I understood our financial position in case he should die."

Matthew: "I did decide that being honest was the better of these two impossibly hard choices. But my great plan didn't always work out. There were times when I didn't feel like talking to anyone, times when I didn't want anybody around. The most horrible moment of my life was the night Aubrey came into my hospital room to tell me a joke: 'Robber: Your money or your life? Storekeeper: Take my life, I'm saving the money for my old age!' It's a good joke, but I couldn't see the humor. It was as if that part of my brain that knows what funny means had died."

Aubrey: "I remember that day, but for me, it was different. I mean my dad is funny. He has a great sense of humor. If he didn't think that joke was a riot, it had to be because he was going through something I couldn't possibly understand. That day I learned to just sit there with him, not saying anything at all. I learned without him even having to tell me that just being there would help him get through another day."

Diana: "It was tough for all of us—I don't want to leave anyone with any Pollyanna impression. But I think it was roughest for Aubrey. He's always had a special spark for Matthew. At the same time, he was only fourteen. That's such an awkward time. Old enough to help out, yet also old enough to want some independence at the same time. The odd weekend, when he did feel like going out with his friends, he'd feel so guilty. Eventually, Matthew himself would tell Aubrey to 'get lost' for the day. They'd wink at each other as Aubrey was on his way out. That relationship must have been made in heaven."

Generally speaking, if a cancer is discovered early, before cells from the primary tumor have had a chance to break off and spread, it is easier to treat. "Once a primary tumor has shed some cells, or metastasized," says Dr. Hasselback, "cancer is more difficult to treat because there is more than one site to worry about."

We can also say that a person who is in good shape—both physically and emotionally—has a better chance of withstanding the terrible months that often go along with cancer treatment.

But there are really no hard-and-fast rules.

You hear about some people whose cancers were *not* diagnosed early surviving for years and years. You see it with all sorts of different cancers. Sometimes, even the doctors are stumped. Why does this happen? Who knows? Some people attribute the ability to survive against all the odds to the immune system. Other people talk about sheer willpower. For some reason, some cancer patients cope with, and respond to, treatment better than others.

On the other hand, some people whose chances of survival seemed excellent when their treatment was finished, discover a couple of years later that their cancer had spread. At the beginning, it looked as if every last cancer cell had been killed off, that there weren't any left alive to spread. In the end, doctors discover that a few cancerous cells, perhaps just one, must have been missed, and it is the metastasis, the second tumor, that eventually causes the person to die.

You hear stories, although not many, about cancer patients who have threatened to give up in the middle of their grueling treatments with radiation or chemicals. You hear that they have said they just can't take it anymore, that dying in peace would be better than living through what, in their experience, is hell.

It's tempting to say as little as possible about the harshness of radiation therapy and chemotherapy, the two most often used forms of cancer treatment other than surgery. It's very tempting, but unfair. It's unfair to the person who is in the middle of treatment and needs understanding, respect, and encouragement to go on. And it is unfair to the family. The emotional pain people can go through watching someone suffer is impossible to describe.

Matthew: "Do people really want to know the details of how much, or how little, you feel like throwing up?" For many cancer patients, a side effect of chemotherapy is nausea and vomiting.

"Do people get bored with you and all your problems? Some days I thought that they did. Even the people who love you are human."

Aubrey: "So he looked a little green at times. That didn't bother me so much, although I must admit I wasn't too thrilled the first time I saw him puke! But to tell the truth, I was happier being there with him than being out with my friends, even during the days when he was so awfully sick."

Matthew: "I didn't want Aubrey to treat me differently, but I *was* different. I needed help with things that a four-year-old could do. There was a period of time when my hands were so weak I couldn't open a jar. I have a picture of myself taken right in the middle of it all. My hair had fallen out from the chemotherapy and I had lost almost forty pounds. I looked like a plucked chicken, although I couldn't joke about it then!"

Aubrey: "Well he's right about that. He looked like hell. Sometimes I worried that he would die from what they were doing to him. How could so terrible a treatment make anyone well? But looking back, I guess the time did fly by. Before we knew it, he was shoveling the food in again just like normal and complaining that he had to lose a few pounds!"

In the end, when treatment is over, most cancer patients who are cured, or at least in remission and looking forward to some productive months, or years, say the tough time was worth it. Almost every one of the former cancer patients I spoke to talks about each extra day of life as a precious gift—*even better than before.* You hear it so often that you have to wonder. . . . If you were to get cancer and survive, would it teach you something about life that you wouldn't regret having learned?

Diana: "I think so, for Matthew. He's changed in a way that is difficult to describe. He notices things, little things he may have thought silly before all this. He has more time to listen to people. He has patience for a story he would have thought boring in the past."

Matthew: "It does sound corny, but I'm alive and even if it's not forever, each day is a joy. If six years ago someone would have told me I'd be counting days as gifts, I would have laughed. What a dumb thing to say!"

Aubrey: "I think that's a fair way of putting it. He was always fabulous to me, but now there's a kind of sensitivity to him that I don't think was there before. . . ."

Many former cancer patients, not only Matthew, talk a lot about the new ways they have learned to relate to people. This doesn't mean that having cancer is a *good* experience. It's terrible. But sometimes it takes a rough time to show you just how much you appreciate the people you love.

Matthew: "I've talked about this with Aubrey quite a bit. He and I go fishing together, just the two of us, every July. We both say that we feel lucky in an odd sort of way. We talk about having shared something special—a negative experience, it's true, but one that has touched us both. It's a fantastic feeling to be able to say to one another, 'God, was I ever scared. Was I ever shaking the whole time.' Scared shitless, is the expression Aubrey always loves to use!"

Aubrey: "All my relationships have changed, not just the one with him. The good part is that I can be really close to people. I think I know what friendship really means. But there's a lousy side too, in a way. The kids I go to school with, the ones who haven't been through something like this . . . there's a barrier between us. It's as if we're living in two different worlds."

Not everyone I spoke to feels as positive as Matthew, Diana, and Aubrey, not everyone at all. A few people said that they were never able to muster the kind of inner strength that got Matthew and his family through. They said they didn't know how to share their feelings with their husbands, wives, and children. They hadn't been particularly open with their feelings *before* cancer struck and couldn't suddenly change the way they related to people.

Some said they just didn't want to "burden anyone else." Others said they weren't "the type to talk." They are as "cured" as Matthew is, at least in the physical sense. But they are still trying to recover the equilibrium that they lost.

In many cases, the family members of these cancer patients said they felt the same way. Their family, which was not particularly close to begin with, fell apart even more. For them, at least for many years, there was little about the experience that was positive, no sharing of fear and of pain. For them, there were just shattered dreams, lost hopes, and the anguish of not knowing what the people you love really think.

It was that way for Jenny, the teenager who, at the beginning of this book, said that knowing more about cancer might help her to cope.

Jenny has no brothers or sisters, just a father, a few aunts and uncles, and a couple of friends. When I talked to her, two years had passed since her mother Anne had had a breast removed because of breast cancer. Anne's radiation therapy and chemotherapy had been over with for more than a year.

It looks as if Anne is as "cured" of breast cancer as Matthew is of leukemia, although, strictly speaking, sixteen years, not five, must pass after treatment is completed before a doctor will pronounce a former breast cancer patient completely cured. In many ways, life has returned to normal for Jenny and her family. Anne has gone back to work. Jenny is doing better in school. And yet, says Jenny, "She still looks so different to me."

Jenny pushes her blonde hair behind her ears when she speaks. Perhaps it is a nervous reaction, as if, even after two years, she is jumpy in the way that Matthew was those first few weeks.

"It's so confusing," she says, "so difficult to explain. For the first time, I see my mother as a separate person, not just as *my* mother. She's no longer the one person I can unload my daily troubles onto. She has burdens of her own.

"Maybe this experience could be a good thing, but she won't let me help. It's almost as if she is trying to be a martyr by coping with it by herself. It makes me angry in a way. I want to help. I've wanted to help since the day it all started. But I want her to ask for my help."

Anne: "I can't talk about this to Jenny. I've never been good at sharing these kinds of things; I wasn't brought up that way. I love Jenny, more than you can imagine, and I'm not stupid. I can sense that she's waiting for me to say something. I used to use the excuse that she's just a little girl, that she couldn't handle it, but now I know I'm the one who's afraid."

Jenny: "The other day I said to her, 'Gee, Mom, if this had been me, I'd really have been scared,' but she just answered, 'Yes, dear.' I got the impression that she was on the verge of saying something, but as usual, she stopped. Perhaps she doesn't want to burden me; she's always been like that. On the other hand, maybe she's okay with the whole thing. I really don't know.

"Yesterday I thought I should just tell her how much I love her and how scared I still am and how we should talk, but I chickened out. I always chicken out. She's the one with the experience in life, so she should be the one to start. Great rationalization, eh! She's never had cancer before either.

"I keep worrying that if I start talking, there will be a flood of emotions. I'm afraid I'll reach a depth that I've never felt before and I won't be able to rise from it. I feel like I'm standing at the edge of a diving board for the first time with my hands over my head, not wanting to go off. I think of every excuse. It drives me crazy."

Anne: "I don't even talk to Jenny's father about it very much. I know it must sound crazy. Being able to talk about life is supposed to be normal in the 1980s. But it's never been that way for me. Jenny's father Bill and I—we don't use words to tell each other how we feel. It doesn't mean we don't care. But I do wish I could give Jenny what she wants. I think about it all the time. It drives me crazy."

Jenny: "Even my dad doesn't say anything about what's happened. He never gets upset. But I think he feels something. Sometimes, when Mom was still in the hospital, I'd come into the house, and he'd be just sitting there, doing nothing, staring into space.

"But whom do I tell all this to? No one I know has ever gone through anything like this. They wouldn't know what I'm talking about. The kids I hang around with would think I'm crazy if I started telling them. And yet, I can't get it out of my mind. I spend a lot of time alone."

Some families are like Matthew's, able to share with each other the pain they are feeling, and it usually helps. The people in families who can talk, and cry, and hold on to each other through the rough days seem to have the easiest of the difficult experiences with cancer.

People in families like Jenny's, where everyone *feels* pain but is too afraid to speak, seem to have a worse time.

Most families, however, are somewhere in between.

Some families start out like Jenny's and slowly, with the help of a psychologist, psychiatrist, social worker, family doctor, member of the clergy, or good friend, learn how to share their emotions. Sometimes it is the parents who realize that they would all do better to talk. Other times it's the kids themselves who muster the courage to make it happen.

In some communities, schools and community centers have developed programs to help. Both the American and Canadian Cancer Societies have one such program called "Coping with Cancer," which anyone—adult or teenager—can join. Some members have cancer, or have had it; others love someone who does. Matthew, for example, leads a group that meets twice a month. "Some people turn to professionals for help and it works for them," he says, "but many people who come to our group say that talking to others who've been there is also a tremendous help."

You can find out about "Coping with Cancer" by calling a local branch of the American or Canadian Cancer Society.

But knowing what may happen, and what to expect, also puts people in a better position to cope with cancer. When all is said and done, when the news that cancer has struck begins to feel real, rather than like a bad dream, knowledge will also help people get through. Once they know the facts about cancer treatment, most people find that they are in a better position to use the rest of their energy to give, or receive, emotional support.

The Diagnosis of Cancer
To make a firm diagnosis of cancer, cells from a person's body must be examined by a doctor called a pathologist whose specialty is identifying disease. There are signs and symptoms that make doctors suspect that a patient has cancer, and they will start looking for cancerous cells. But a final diagnosis cannot be made until cells are actually

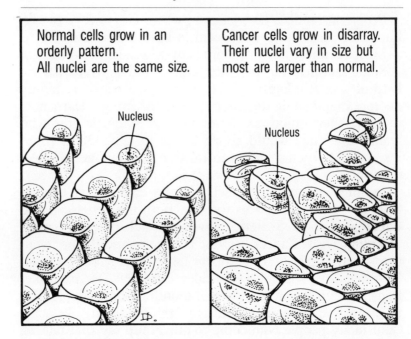

Normal cells grow in an orderly pattern. All nuclei are the same size.

Nucleus

Cancer cells grow in disarray. Their nuclei vary in size but most are larger than normal.

Nucleus

studied in a lab under a microscope, and proven to be cancerous.

Most of the time, there is a tumor—which may or may not be cancerous—whose cells can be examined. The exception is leukemia, the type of cancer Matthew had. Because leukemia is spread throughout a system, the bloodstream, there is no actual tumor. Instead, the bone marrow, where the diseased blood cells are produced, must be examined for cancerous cells.

Most tumors do not turn out to be cancerous. Eight out of ten breast tumors, for example, are "benign," or noncancerous. Benign tumors are removed, and that is the end of it. They do not metastasize, or spread, like cancerous or "malignant" tumors. They can be dangerous, but only because they sometimes grow, getting in the way of other vital organs and tissue.

Getting a sample of cells to study is called taking a biopsy. Sometimes the whole tumor is removed, and this is called an "excisional" biopsy. Other times, only a section of the tumor is cut away, and this is called an "incisional" biopsy. In the case of leukemia, a bit of bone marrow is "aspirated," or sucked up, with a long, thin needle. The pathologist uses a microscope, as well as blood tests, to determine whether the marrow is producing cancerous or normal white blood cells.

Sometimes, as was the case with Anne's breast cancer, doctors start looking for a tumor because something unusual turns up during a routine checkup.

Other times, the patient is the one who becomes suspicious. Like Matthew, he or she notices one of the ten basic signs that the American and Canadian Cancer Societies warn people to watch out for. They are:

1. A sore that does not heal.
2. A change in a mole or wart.
3. The sudden appearance of a lump or a bump.
4. A cough that continues to worsen for several weeks, or blood in the sputum.
5. Vaginal discharge or bleeding other than during a menstrual period.
6. A *change* in one's bowel habits: constipation or diarrhea.
7. Blood in the urine.
8. Persistent pain.
9. Persistent fever.
10. Unexplainable weakness, or weight loss, or exhaustion over a period of time.

It is particularly sad when a person notices one of these signs or symptoms but, out of fear, perhaps, delays going for a medical checkup. Too many doctors have stories of cancer patients who could have been helped, if only treatment had been started earlier.

Sometimes a tumor is relatively easy to find. Other times it is more difficult to locate.

When a tumor is accessible, taking a biopsy is usually easy. For instance, it is almost always a simple procedure to obtain a sample of cells from a suspicious-looking tumor on the cervix (the entrance to the womb), and taking a biopsy from a suspicious-looking skin tumor is usually simple as well. These procedures can generally be performed in a doctor's office with only a local anesthetic.

Having a bit of bone marrow aspirated requires a brief stay in hospital. The procedure is usually painful, but only for a moment. The skin is first anesthetized, then a long syringe, or needle, is inserted into the marrow of a bone—usually a hipbone, but sometimes a breastbone. Finally, a small amount of the marrow is sucked up. The entire procedure takes only a few minutes.

In Anne's case, the cancerous breast tumor was easy to locate, but more difficult to biopsy. Her doctor, who was performing a routine checkup, could feel the lump, which was growing in one of Anne's breasts. But to get a sample of cells, Anne had to have a general anesthetic and then a minor surgical procedure. While the pathologist in the lab determined that the tumor was actually cancerous, Anne remained under general anesthesia, and then, during the same operation, the cancerous breast was "resected," or removed.

Other times, when a tumor is growing in an organ such as the kidney, pancreas, or liver (which are all located deep within the body), a major surgical procedure must be performed to obtain cells for a biopsy.

But most of the time surgery is not required. Because of recent advances in diagnostic methods, tumors in many organs can be located and biopsied in one simple procedure called endoscopy. An endoscope is a long, thin instrument made of flexible fibers, called fiber optics, which can actually transmit light. There is also a pair of tiny "scissors" at the end of most endoscopes. Endoscopes can be inserted into many organs of the body: the lungs, stomach, colon, uterus, and bladder are some of the organs that are now accessible through endoscopy.

In fact, although it is never done, a doctor technically could insert one endoscope through the mouth into the stomach, and another through the rectum into the intestinal tract, and they could meet in the middle.

Once an endoscope is inside an organ, the doctor turns on the light and inspects the area. If a tumor is visible, the trigger is pressed and snip! A piece of tissue is snared, carefully withdrawn, and sent to the lab for examination.

There are many types of endoscopes. Colonoscopes, for example, are used to examine the entire length of the colon; gastroscopes are used to examine the stomach; cystoscopes are used to examine the bladder.

Many of the cancer patients I spoke to had been terrified of having a biopsy taken with an endoscope. They had heard stories about how painful it was to get a sample of lung, stomach, or colon tissue by this method. Ten years ago, this was true. The endoscopes that were used then were not flexible and it was often painful to insert the instrument, especially if the tumor was deep within the organ. This is no longer the case. Today, endoscopy is sometimes uncomfortable, but rarely painful.

To get a biopsy from a lung tumor, for example, a type of endoscope called a bronchoscope is used. The doctor sprays an anesthetic into the throat and then gently inserts the flexible tube down the throat right into a bronchus, or airway, to a lung. Once the instrument is in place, the light goes on, and the tissue that lines the airway is examined. Most lung tumors develop in a bronchus.

If there is a tumor, the doctor will remove a sample of tissue and place a tiny piece between two pieces of glass for protection, then send it to a lab. There, the pathologist will examine the cells and make the decision: are the cells cancerous? And, if they are, exactly what kind of cancer is it?

When cancer is being diagnosed, other tests are usually performed as well. Some of them can determine whether or not the first tumor has spread.

The blood, for example, is chemically tested to see if it contains the normal amount of white blood cells, red blood cells, enzymes, proteins, and minerals.

For most kinds of cancer, the X-ray is an important test. Only a few years ago, normal X-rays—a beam of X-rays and film much like the kind used in a camera—were generally used. Over the past decade, however, the whole field of X-ray technology has been changing.

In some hospitals, CT scanners (sometimes called CAT, which stands for computer aided tomography, scanners) are used to take pictures of small areas deep within the body. The pictures—paper-thin "slices" of organs—that CT scanners provide are incredible. Already CT scanners are taking the place of many of the more complicated and uncomfortable tests.

Another new way of getting pictures similar to those provided by CT scanners is through "NMR," nuclear magnetic resonance. These pictures can be taken without exposing the patient to any radiation at all.

Sometimes, just before an X-ray is taken, the patient is given an injection of a dye which acts as a contrast, making whatever the doctor is looking for stand out better. These dyes are harmless and painless. They are sometimes used when ordinary X-rays are taken, and before some CT scans.

"Bone scanners" work on the principle that tumor cells react differently than normal cells to radioactive isotopes that are injected into the blood. During a bone scan, tumor cells—which divide more quickly than normal cells—show up as "hot spots." This is a fast, completely painless method of pinpointing a bone tumor that is sometimes no more than a centimeter in diameter. Once the exact location of a tumor is known, it is much easier to obtain a biopsy to determine if it is malignant or benign.

If there is fluid in the chest cavity, in the abdomen, or in a joint, some of it will be extracted and examined for cancerous cells. First, a local anesthetic is injected, then a long, but extremely thin needle is inserted. A bit of fluid is then suctioned out with little discomfort.

Sometimes some of the fluid in the spinal canal is examined as well. A "spinal tap" used to be a scary and uncomfortable experience. But these days, with better equipment and a tiny needle to freeze the area before the larger one is inserted, a pinprick is all that most people feel.

Once the question, "Is it cancer?" has been affirmed by the pathologist, the next step will be to decide exactly what kind of cancer it is, how far it has progressed, and what the treatment should be.

The Terms That Are Used

Cancer can develop in almost all the body's organs. The heart, whose cells do not reproduce after maturity, is a notable exception.

Physicians divide the many different types of cancer into four main groups: carcinomas, leukemias, lymphomas (which include myelomas), and sarcomas.

Carcinomas, such as lung cancer, breast cancer, and cancer of the colon, rectum, cervix, and stomach, are by far the most common.

Carcinomas begin in epithelial cells. These are the cells that line the inside and outside surfaces of the various organs of the body. Cancerous tumors of the cervix, for example, begin in the epithelial cells that line the organ's *external* surface; cancerous tumors of the colon, on the other hand, begin in the epithelial cells that line the *internal* surface of that organ.

Leukemias are cancers of various types of leukocytes, or white blood cells that are produced in the bone marrow.

Lymphomas are cancers of the lymphocytes, the white blood cells of the lymphatic system. Myelomas are cancers of particular white blood cells called plasma cells. Plasma cells start off as B lymphocytes and then move into the lymphatic system, where they mature further into plasma cells. They are stored in bone marrow.

Sarcomas are cancers of mesodermal cells: bone, muscle, cartilage, tendon, and ligament cells which form supportive and connective tissues.

Cancers that begin in the brain are so different from any other type of cancer that they are usually discussed separately.

Cancer cells usually go through a stage—called precancer—during which they appear abnormal when they are examined under a microscope, but not so abnormal that pathologists consider them cancerous. Sometimes precancerous cells can be detected, but not because they exhibit symptoms. They are detected through mass-screening programs, such as the Pap test, which are now performed in the hope of detecting precancerous cells of the cervix. The cells of the cervix, for example, go through precancerous changes, called dysplasia, before cancer actually occurs. Precancerous changes sometimes reverse themselves with no treatment at all. And even when they do not, they are relatively easy to cure.

If a precancerous cell does progress into a cancer cell, it will usually develop on the surface of the organ. At that point, it is called an "in situ" or early cancer. Like precancerous conditions, early cancers are usually relatively easy to treat successfully.

However, as it begins to grow, a cancer tumor will invade the tissue on which it has developed. At this point, it is referred to as an "invasive cancer." But as long as the cells remain in a single mass—that is, as long as no cells have metastasized from the primary tumor—the cancer is said to be "localized."

Then metastasis begins. First, a few cells break off from the primary tumor and travel through the blood vessels or the lymphatic channels to other parts of the body.

Sometimes the cells that move into the lymphatic system get trapped for a while in the bean-shaped lymph nodes that are found at different points along this system. Usually it is the first few shed cells that get trapped by a lymph node, and, more often than not, the nodes are those that are nearby—that is, *in the region of* the original tumor. When this happens, the spreading process is slowed down for a while, and the cancer is labeled "invasive cancer with regional involvement." This is what Anne's breast cancer was labeled.

If there is no treatment, or if treatment is unsuccessful, the cancer cells will almost always spread to more distant parts of the body, where they will grow into "secondary tumors." This is "advanced" cancer. There are always exceptions but, generally speaking, it is almost impossible to cure cancer once it has reached the advanced stage. Most people with advanced cancer die within five years.

One of the reasons why the death rate from cancer is so high is that cancer is usually not detected until it has reached at least the invasive, and frequently the advanced stage. This is often nobody's fault. It's just that there are frequently no symptoms—no pain, or anything suspicious to notice—while cancer is still at an early stage. The only thing that doctors and researchers can stress is this: if someone notices anything suspicious, any of the symptoms listed on page 65, he or she should be examined by a doctor immediately. Cancer generally becomes deadly only when it has invaded an organ or when it has spread, and often it can be detected before this occurs.

The name doctors give to a particular type of cancer depends on where it has begun. If a cancer tumor begins in a breast, for example, it is always called breast cancer. It is still called breast cancer if it spreads to another part of the body, say, the lungs. Even if the breast has been removed, and a new tumor develops in a lung from a shed breast tumor cell many years later, it would still be referred to as breast cancer. Technically, doctors would call it a "breast cancer which has metastasized to the lung." The breast tumor would have been the primary tumor and the lung tumor would be a secondary tumor. This makes sense when you recall that the cancer cells which have metastasized to the lung to form a secondary tumor, will still be *breast* cells, rather than lung cells.

Cancer Treatment
There are basically three types of cancer treatment: surgery, radiation therapy, and chemotherapy. Often a combination of two of these three treatments is used. And sometimes, as was the case with the treatment for Anne's breast cancer, all three are used.

Researchers are also constantly seeking ways of improving these treatments. New forms of radiation have been developed. New drugs, and better ways of using the established formulas for existing drugs, are always being found. Completely new methods are being developed as well. Immunotherapy, for example, which tries to stimulate the body's immune system, is one. How long it will take before these new treatments are available to all cancer patients is impossible to say, but cancer research has never looked as promising as it does today.

Surgery
Many things must be taken into account before surgery is chosen as a treatment for cancer. First of all, there must be a tumor. The entire bloodstream, for example, can't be surgically removed, and so surgery for leukemia is out of the question. Second, the tumor must be able to be reached, and it must be in an organ that can be resected, or removed, without causing death. A breast tumor can be resected; a breast is not essential to life. A liver tumor cannot be removed. By the time a cancerous liver tumor is detected, it has usually invaded the organ. For surgery to be successful, the entire liver would have to be removed, and a person can't survive without a liver.

If the conditions are favorable and the patient is not too old or too ill to withstand surgery, the tumor will usually be removed. Working ever so gently to avoid knocking off any cells that could spread, the surgeon will cut away all the cancerous tissue that can be seen, as well as a margin of surrounding normal tissue.

Normal tissue is removed as a preventive measure, mostly because cancer tumors don't grow in tight lumps. Like a patch of crabgrass growing in a lawn, cancer tumors have root-like projections that branch off from the main body. Remember the crab? It is important that the surgeon remove enough tissue for a safety margin. If any cells were to be left behind—technically, if one cancer cell were left behind—a new tumor could possibly develop.

Surgery has certainly changed over the past couple of decades. There are better antibiotics—the drugs used to control infection—and better anesthetics that don't leave patients feeling quite so wiped out.

Surgeons have also learned to perform cancer operations in a much more delicate way. Breast surgery, for example, has changed significantly. In the past, the tumor the rest of the breast, the muscle underneath the breast, and the glands nearby—the lymph nodes—were all removed. Today, disfiguring "radical mastectomies" are not performed nearly as often.

Anne had a breast and a number of lymph nodes removed. In her case, enough tissue was able to be saved so that a "prosthesis," or breast mold, could be fitted easily. Anyone who is unaware that Anne has had a mastectomy would certainly not realize it from looking at her, "even when I am wearing an evening gown," she says.

"Radical surgery for breast cancer," says Dr. Hasselback, "is performed less than half the time. Instead, if a surgeon feels that any cancer cells have already metastasized from the main tumor, either radiation therapy or chemotherapy, or both, will be used to 'mop them up.' "

Radiation Therapy
Since radiation affects any cell that is in the middle of dividing, it ought to affect more cancer cells than normal cells. Why? Because cancer cells, if you recall, divide far more frequently than normal cells. This was the reasoning behind the development of radiation therapy for the treatment of cancer, and the reason why it is still used today.

Radiation doesn't exactly *kill* cancer cells. Rather, it damages the DNA in the nucleus of these cells, and when its DNA is damaged, a cell cannot divide. When cancer cells can no longer divide, they die. Therefore, instead of growing larger, a cancerous tumor that is bombarded with radiation will shrink.

As with surgery, radiation therapy has certain limitations. For one thing, it can only be used on an organ that stays fixed. Most of us are unaware of the fact that the colon, for example, is an organ that keeps moving around. Waving throughout the abdomen as it goes about its business of digesting food and moving waste, the colon is like a moving target. A radiology oncologist can't aim radiation at a target that moves, and so cannot use this form of treatment for cancer of the colon.

Some organs are able to tolerate more radiation than

others. The cells of the pancreas, for example, can handle much more radiation than can the cells of the kidneys. The kidneys are located in front of the pancreas, however, and to shrink a cancer tumor of the pancreas, a radiologist would have to use more radiation than the cells of the kidney could withstand. That's one reason radiation cannot be used to shrink a tumor of the pancreas.

Radiation therapy works best on a fixed tumor, or group of tumors, spread over a large accessible area. Hodgkin's disease, a type of lymphoma which usually involves a group of lymph nodes, is an example of a type of cancer for which radiation therapy works especially well.

Radiation therapy has changed significantly over the years. In the 1920s and 30s, it was all but useless for any type of cancer other than skin cancer. It's not that it didn't work; it did. But regular X-rays were not very strong, and in order to deliver enough radiation to shrink a tumor deep within the body, so much had to be used that normal tissue was extensively damaged. The skin was burned, and all the tissue between the skin and the cancer tumor was damaged as well. For that reason radiation had to be confined to tumors growing in the skin itself.

Then, in 1956, cobalt radiation was discovered. Cobalt is a metal that can be made radioactive, and the rays it delivers are much stronger than regular X-rays. Using cobalt machines, radiologists were able to deliver "megavoltage" radiation to tumors deep within the body, without damaging organs in between.

Sometimes tumors can be completely destroyed by radiation, and the patient can be cured with no other treatment. Other times a tumor can be shrunk sufficiently so that curative surgery becomes possible. And, in still other cases, radiation is used in conjunction with chemotherapy.

Radiation is now being used in other ways as well. Sometimes "needles" made of radioactive material are inserted directly into a tumor and then removed after the treatment is finished. This is a fabulous advance for tumors of the head or neck, which, if treated surgically, would leave very severe scars.

The advances in radiation therapy have also been exciting for patients with certain other specific types of cancer. A rare type of eye cancer called retinoblastoma, which strikes young children, can now often be cured with radiation therapy. Because surgery can be avoided, these children do not lose the use of an eye.

The same type of advance has been made using radiation therapy for cancer of the larynx, or voice box. In the days when this type of cancer could only be treated by surgery, the entire larynx had to be removed, and patients lost their ability to speak. With radiation therapy there is no need for surgery, and many former cancer-of-the-larynx patients are living totally normal lives.

Recently, doctors have been successful at radiating the entire body for certain types of leukemia and lymphoma.

Even when a cancer has progressed too far for a cure to be possible, radiation can sometimes be used. Some types of tumors can be shrunk enough to prolong the patient's life for several years. For advanced cancers, radiation can sometimes be used to relieve pain when a tumor is pressing on a bone or on other tissue.

Although radiation therapy has advanced by leaps and bounds, it is still difficult for cancer patients to cope with in certain ways.

People who receive radiation therapy to their heads still lose their hair, just as they did several decades ago. The cells which attach the hair to the head—called hair follicles—divide much more quickly than most normal cells. Because of this, the DNA in these cells is destroyed by radiation in the same way as the DNA in cancer cells. Without DNA, the hair cells cannot reproduce, and the hair falls out.

While hair loss is emotionally upsetting, it is not a terrible price to pay in exchange for life. For one thing, hair grows back as soon as treatment is finished. The other side effects of radiation therapy are worse.

The cells that line the stomach and intestines are also fast-dividing, and so radiation to the abdomen causes severe nausea, vomiting, and diarrhea.

The white blood cells, which protect the body from infection, have an extremely short life span—only eight hours, in fact. During radiation therapy their DNA is destroyed, and they are unable to divide to replace cells that have died. For this reason, people undergoing radiation therapy have too few white blood cells to perform the important job of fighting off infection. Fortunately, researchers have developed better antibiotics to help combat infection.

The numbers of platelets, which protect against bleeding, often get low as well, and people bruise easily and find that injuries don't heal.

These side effects last only as long as the radiation treatments continue, and they are not nearly as severe as they once were.

RADIATION THERAPY—NEW RESEARCH
The first studies on humans using a variation of radiation therapy—called pion beam therapy—are beginning to show some extraordinary results for tumors located deep within the body. This is particularly exciting since conventional cobalt therapy has proved to be virtually useless for cancers of the brain, pancreas, and bladder.

Pions are the subatomic, glue-like particles that hold together, or bind, the neutrons, protons, and electrons contained in the nuclei of all cells. Now, pions can be extracted by machines called cyclotrons. When the Los Alamos, New Mexico, center (where the atomic bomb was developed) was closed a few years ago, only two centers that work with pions were left—one in Switzerland, the other in Canada. Dr. Gabriel Lam, a research biophysicist at the B.C. Cancer Research Centre in Vancouver, British Columbia, has been working with pions on Canada's $50-million cyclotron machine for ten years.

"Cyclotrons extract pions by breaking apart the neutrons, protons, and electrons in cells' nuclei, which causes them to release a pion," he explains. "But it wasn't until the 1970s that enough pions were able to be extracted to make experiments on cancer tumors possible."

Pions are delivered to cancer tumors by an electromagnetic beam. When the pions hit the cancer cells, they release energy—like a depth charge—and the cancer cells are killed. Pion beams do very little damage to the tissue that they pass through on their way to cancer tumors, and they are also strong enough to reach tumors that are too deep for cobalt radiation.

Unfortunately, it will still be years before pion beam radiation therapy is available to most cancer patients. One of the biggest obstacles in getting this type of therapy into general use is the price. The type of cyclotrons required by hospitals to extract pions don't cost $50 million, but they do cost between $5 and $10 million each.

A further variation on radiation therapy which Dr. Lam is beginning to investigate is neutron beam therapy. Neutrons are also subatomic particles, and they too can be extracted from the nuclei of cells with a cyclotron machine. Whether or not they will prove useful in the treatment of cancer remains to be seen. Dr. Lam believes that neutron beams will be effective for many more types of cancer than are pion beams, which are only useful for deep tumors. The other advantage to neutron beam radiation therapy is that the type of cyclotron machine required to produce neutrons costs less—approximately $2.5 million.

Chemotherapy
The most exciting advances in cancer treatment have been made with chemotherapy. Over the years, cancer-killing chemicals have saved, or at least extended, the lives of tens of thousands of cancer patients around the world.

Chemotherapy began during World War II when a physician from the University of Chicago, Charles Huggins, filled a syringe with the female hormone estrogen and injected it into the bloodstream of a man with cancer of the prostate. Within a few weeks the growth of the man's tumor slowed down, and, for the first time in history, a drug had been used effectively in the battle against cancer.

The beauty of treating cancer with chemicals is that drugs can travel throughout the bloodstream. With surgery, only the tumor itself can be removed. With radiation, except in a few circumstances when it is used on the whole body, the beam can only be aimed at one specific spot. That's fine if the cancer tumor has not spread. But too often at least a few cells have already metastasized from the main tumor by the time surgery or radiation therapy is performed. These shed cells may have already formed a "micro-metastasis," a tiny secondary tumor, some distance away. A long time may pass, years perhaps, before a micro-metastasis actually grows into a secondary tumor that is large enough to be detected. But because chemotherapy travels throughout the body via the bloodstream, many cancer patients who receive this kind of treatment are now being cured.

In the late 1940s, a group of researchers at Yale University in Connecticut began to expand on Dr. Huggins' experiments by making use of a chance disaster. During World War II, the U.S. was trying to develop chemicals for use in warfare when some mustard gas, with which they were experimenting, exploded. The Yale scientists read that the people killed in the explosion had died because the gas had damaged their white blood cells.

The Yale researchers theorized that it might be possible to use a similar chemical to fight lymphoma, cancer of the lymph system. The theory was logical since the problem with lymphoma patients is that they have too many white blood cells.

They tried nitrogen mustard, a chemical related to mustard gas, on a patient with cancer of the lymphatic system. Sure enough, the cancerous white blood cells disappeared, although only for a short time. Today, more than thirty years later, the drug is still used—although more skillfully—to treat Hodgkin's disease, a specific type of lymphoma.

At about the same time, another major advance using chemicals was made. Dr. Sidney Farber, the doctor for whom the world-famous Sidney Farber Cancer Institute in Boston is named, was responsible. He realized that the cancer cells of children with leukemia grew faster if the children were given large amounts of a certain vitamin B.

If a drug could be made to *interfere* with the body's use

of this vitamin, Dr. Farber speculated, it might inhibit the cancer cells as well.

In his lab, Dr. Farber came up with a drug called "aminopterin." For ten out of the sixteen dying children he first tried it on, aminopterin brought successful, although temporary, results.

Because of pioneers like these, a huge program to develop chemotherapy was started in the 1950s in the United States. It began with five million dollars that Congress allocated to the NCI, the National Cancer Institute, which is the branch of the American Cancer Society that funds cancer research. Since the program was started, approximately forty anti-cancer drugs have been discovered or created.

Chemotherapy is being used increasingly for cancers such as leukemia, which cannot be treated by surgery. Doctors are achieving some excellent results, especially with children. In the beginning, only one drug was generally tried for each type of cancer. Now, a combination of drugs is generally used.

Some of these drugs stop cancer cells from making the DNA they require in order to begin the first stage of cell division. Others work by paralyzing the cancer cells while they are in the middle of dividing. And still others, like methotrexate, which was an advancement on Dr. Farber's aminopterin, trick cancer cells by masquerading as vitamins.

Methotrexate is like the mythological Trojan horse that looked like a horse but contained a belly full of soldiers. To the cancer cell, methotrexate *looks* like vitamin B, but when the cancer cell absorbs this "vitamin," it soon finds that it has taken in something which it cannot digest. Cancer cells literally choke on cancer drugs like methotrexate.

Today chemotherapy is often used in conjunction with surgery or radiation therapy, and sometimes with both. In many cases chemotherapy is started almost as soon as a cancer patient comes off the operating table, or a tumor has been shrunk by radiation.

Why wait to see if a metastasis shows up, when chemotherapy can be used right away? The hope is that if a few shed cells from the primary tumor have been missed, they will be killed by chemotherapy *before* they have a chance to grow into secondary tumors. This type of chemotherapy treatment is called "adjuvant chemotherapy." When it is successful, a second tumor never develops. Over the past few years, adjuvant chemotherapy has been used for breast cancer patients like Anne. It is too soon to know for sure, but oncologists such as Dr. Hasselback believe that more and more successes are going to be seen because of it.

That is the beauty of chemotherapy, but there is an ugly side to it as well. Almost all the drugs that are used to fight cancer are poisonous. They cause worse side effects than radiation therapy or surgery.

When having radiation therapy to their heads, patients lose their hair. All chemotherapy drugs, however, travel throughout the bloodstream. Almost all the drugs affect the blood vessels of the scalp where the hair follicle cells are located. Therefore, *most* chemotherapy patients lose their hair. As with radiation therapy, hair grows back when the chemotherapy is over, but hair loss is not the worst side effect of this type of treatment.

Nausea and vomiting are often a side effect of the chemicals that are used. As well, the DNA of the fast-dividing cells that line the mouth and the throat is damaged; for this reason some patients lose their sense of taste and the ability to swallow without extreme discomfort.

Matthew remembers those first weeks of intensive chemotherapy: "I was on a very heavy dose of several drugs for five days; they must have mixed up that devil concoction in a blender! Then they let me off for a few weeks to recover. At the end of those three weeks, they did another bone marrow test to see if I was in 'remission,' if all the cancer cells appeared to have been killed. The drugs had worked; I *was* in remission. But God, during those first five days there were times when I'd be throwing up every twenty minutes. Some nights I didn't believe I had the courage to go on."

Diana: "In some ways, looking back, I think those days took almost as much out of us as him. You feel so powerless when someone you love is in pain, and there is nothing you can do."

Aubrey: "You'd look at him in the morning and you'd think he'd been through a war. But once those first five days were over, it wasn't quite as bad. You could see his strength coming back, little by little."

One of the greatest problems for people who are undergoing chemotherapy is weight loss. Food is not appealing when you can't taste it and when you feel nauseated constantly. Some people find that eating a large number of small meals each day, rather than three large ones, is helpful. Other people try to keep their weight up by snacking on tasty, high-calorie treats, such as milk shakes. Most people try to avoid fatty foods, which are particularly hard to digest. An entire booklet, advising people on how to cope with weight loss and nutrition while on chemotherapy, has been published by the American Cancer Society.

Matthew: "During those first five days I ate nothing. Nothing! Then, I started on a few things. Potato chips, I loved potato chips. Crazy, eh? Most cancer patients find them too rich, too hard to digest. But that was one of the first things I could eat when my five-day journey was over."

Aubrey: "I brought him his first bag. Onion-flavored! It was funny to watch him. Before that he'd sort of push his food around, trying to hide things under pieces of lettuce so we'd think he was eating. I used to do that when Mom cooked liver. But you should have seen him with those chips. Boy, what a pig!"

Some cancer patients have found that smoking marijuana helps with the nauseating side effects of chemotherapy. For years many people, except the police who made a few arrests, did not take the idea of marijuana for cancer patients very seriously. Then a number of doctors told their patients that they would go to court on their behalf if they were arrested for smoking marijuana, and more people began to take the risk.

Eventually, a pharmaceutical company created a marijuana-like pill called Nabalone, which is synthesized from the part of the marijuana plant that seems to calm people. Some people insist that it has been a lifesaver. Others say Nabalone does nothing much for them at all. A few people say that it has its own side effects, such as making time seem as if it is passing more slowly. These people usually say that Nabalone just makes them feel worse.

Matthew: "They gave me Nabalone during those first five days. At first I liked it. I felt, you know, high."

Diana: "I must admit, I had to laugh. Most mothers worry about their *kids* taking drugs! I never thought I'd see Matthew high as a kite."

Aubrey: "You should have seen him. One time I walked in and he was in the bathtub singing. I mean, talk about role reversals—my father, stoned out of his tree."

Matthew: "A couple of days later, the effects sort of wore off. I know other people for whom Nabalone has worked better. I just became more aware of my stress."

Chemotherapy, like radiation therapy, also affects the normal blood cells which, like cancer cells, divide frequently. Patients become extremely tired and susceptible to infections. Sometimes their gums bleed, and they bruise more easily than normal.

What's worse is that, for the past few years, oncologists have been giving patients stronger doses of drugs for longer periods of time, in the hope of killing every last cancer cell that may have escaped surgery or radiation therapy.

Each phase of chemotherapy is planned to fit the patient's exact needs. How a patient reacts to the drugs, of course, is also taken into account. Generally, a course of therapy is planned in two parts. The first part is designed to kill the bulk of the cancer cells, and is sometimes repeated. The second part is referred to as "maintenance therapy."

The first phase is sometimes like Matthew's program. Very strong drugs are administered for a five-day period, called a "course." There may be several courses over a number of months. This phase is designed to put the patient into remission and is the roughest part. Matthew was lucky. He went into remission after the first five-day course. His two additional courses, one in February, the next in

March, were given for added protection, in case some cancer cells had been missed during the first course.

Other cancer patients get the first phase once a week for a month, either all at once or over a period of a couple of days. Some are on drugs steadily for a month, getting one type one week, and another type the next. How a patient reacts to treatment depends on what drugs are used and the individual's ability to cope with them, and with stress.

Maintenance therapy can sometimes last as long as a couple of years. The drugs used during this second phase are rarely as strong as during the first phase. Most cancer patients can live normal lives during the second phase of chemotherapy.

Some maintenance therapy patients come into the hospital for a few days each month and take pills or injections at home in between. The luckiest are able to take all the drugs they need in tablet form. Some people do suffer mild side effects, but the emotional stress associated with wondering if the chemicals will keep the cancer in remission is usually far worse than any physical discomfort they have.

Matthew: "That second part, it's true, wasn't so bad. It went on for two years. I felt awful at times—nauseated and tired. But the fear was far worse than the physical symptoms. It was like a humming in the background, a radio that was never quite turned off. Secretly, I called it my background Muzak, and every time I had to go in for another blood test to ensure that I was still in remission, the volume of my Muzak went up. Diana and I tried not to lay too much of that on the kids. But I can remember buying Sol a little two-wheeler with training wheels at the end of that first year. At that point, I wasn't convinced that I'd see him ride that bike by himself. I don't worry about it all that much anymore."

Diana: "Matthew shared most of his fears with me and I tried to absorb them. We're an open family but by that time I didn't see the point of laying this burden onto the kids. . . . I remember that little two-wheeler, watching Matthew from the living room window, screwing on the training wheels with tears in his eyes. I knew what he was thinking."

Aubrey: "They think we didn't know. But after a while, we got to know the schedule. Four days before he went in for a blood test, Dad would get a bit cranky. The day before, they both were a wreck. But it didn't last. I don't think I worry about it all that often anymore."

Oncologists hope that the side effects of these stronger and longer-lasting courses of treatment will be balanced on the positive side by better results. But for many of the newer drug combinations the results are still unknown. "It takes years, sometimes," says Dr. Hasselback, "to be certain that a metastasis is not going to show up. Breast cancer patients are not considered totally cured for approximately sixteen years after treatment. Leukemia patients must wait five years for a completely clean bill of health. Lymphoma patients must wait eight years, and for most types of carcinoma, five years are necessary before a patient is considered cured. Part of the anguish is waiting to see."

Matthew: "I guess now it's mostly Christmas and birthdays that make me a little edgy. I get a sort of bittersweet feeling. It means much more to me to be here for another year. But you know, rare as it is, leukemia patients off treatment for six years have gone out of remission before."

Aubrey: "I guess it crosses all of our minds at Christmas. Birthdays too, especially his. But we'll make it. I know someone who has been cured of leukemia for fifteen years. I think it helps that we sometimes still talk about it. The fact that we could always talk about it, when we needed to, is what really got us through."

Immunotherapy
Cancer researchers called immunologists are working to learn more about the possibilities of the latest development in cancer treatment to date: immunotherapy. Until a few years ago "immunology" sparked very little interest among the public. Then someone got wind of the research being done with a substance called interferon, and, like wildfire spreading, the news hit the stands.

Other exciting areas of immunology are being studied as

well: bone marrow transplantation, monoclonal antibodies, and anti-cancer vaccines are all beginning to yield exciting preliminary results.

INTERFERON

Interferon probably took the public by storm in part because when it was first used we were all eager for a little uplifting news in the area of cancer research. Also, the name interferon seems so positive, so appropriate for a fighter against cancer. When it first became possible to make sufficient quantities of interferon in the lab for testing purposes, articles with snazzy headlines began to hit the news.

Interferon, said some, is going to become "the new Wonder Drug." It is going to be the new multipurpose chemical that will kick the body's immune system back into gear. What's more, because interferon is a *natural* chemical, it is going to do all this with no dreadful side effects. And it is going to do it all almost overnight.

It didn't happen quite that way. Investigating a drug like interferon takes years of painstaking research. Unfortunately, much of the media neglected to mention this minor detail.

So far, interferon has certainly caused cancer tumors to shrink, but it has not done it any better than many of the other chemical therapies.

Why not? Part of the reason has to do with the fact that science still lacks a lot of knowledge about the immune system itself. Does cancer suppress the immune system so much that nothing can get it back into working order? Some studies show that carcinogens like cigarette smoke do interfere with the functioning of the immune system to some degree, but in truth, scientists don't really know.

Maybe cancer interferes with the immune system *progressively* as it takes over the body. Interferon has only been used on patients with advanced cancer. Perhaps by that time it is too late. Or perhaps interferon stimulates only NK cells to work harder than normal. Since NK cells kill only viruses, it could be that interferon will only turn out to be an effective drug for those few types of cancer that are caused by viruses.

Once some of these questions are answered, more information about interferon and other types of immunological treatments will emerge.

We have to hope that the press will learn to look at these experiments with some restraint. This type of research takes time and we must remember this—as difficult as it is to remain patient when someone we love needs immediate treatment.

In any case, the part about interferon being natural and free of side effects is true. For this reason, and because we continue to hope, researchers will press ahead with experiments on interferon and other types of chemicals that might stimulate the immune system to fight against cancer.

VACCINES

Vaccines that would prevent cancer from developing are also being investigated. Experiments on animals have shown that vaccines can be effective in preventing certain rare types of cancers that are caused by viruses. Perhaps someday a vaccine will be developed to prevent some types of cancer in humans.

BONE MARROW TRANSPLANTATION

A couple of new areas of immunology do look promising, however. One of them has to do with bone marrow transplantation.

When a person has leukemia, the bone marrow produces cancerous cells. Certain anti-cancer drugs, such as the ones given to Matthew, can sometimes kill these cancerous cells, and the patient goes into remission. At that point, the cells produced by the bone marrow are healthy.

At other times chemotherapy is not successful. In certain circumstances, usually when the patient is under forty and otherwise in good health, a bone marrow transplant is considered. A donor whose cells have the same HLA markers as the cancer patient's cells must be found to provide marrow for transplantation. If the markers are different, the cancer patient's immune system will perceive the donated marrow as foreign and will not accept it. Often a brother or a sister of the cancer patient is a suitable donor. Cells from siblings are studied genetically, and if the HLA markers do match, healthy bone marrow is extracted from the donor's hipbone. This marrow is then injected into the cancer patient's bloodstream, in much the same way as blood is transfused. (If you're interested in more detail, see page 167.) Since the HLA markers are the same, the chances of the cancer patient accepting the transplanted bone marrow are good. If it is accepted, the cancer patient will be able to produce healthy blood cells.

Bone marrow transplantation is, however, a risky procedure. Prior to the transplant, all of the cancer patient's bone marrow—and, with luck, all the cancer cells in it—must be destroyed by strong drugs. At that point, no one can say for sure if the transplanted marrow will be accepted, and if it isn't, the patient will die.

In a few centers in the U.S., another type of experiment is being tried on leukemia patients for whom chemotherapy has already been successful. When the patient is in remission, bone marrow is extracted and frozen. The hope is that the leukemia patient will be able to become his or her own donor, *if and when* there is a relapse. Since the transplant would be from the patient's own body, the HLA markers would, of course, be the same, and there would be no question of rejection. The one worry would be that a few stray cancer cells may have been frozen in the marrow inadvertently. More research in this area must be done.

MONOCLONAL ANTIBODIES
The other area of immunological research has to do with cells called "monoclonal antibodies." This research is not quite as advanced as the research on bone marrow transplantation, but initial experiments look promising.

If scientists end up with the positive results that the preliminary research is indicating, the dreadful side effects of chemotherapy will become dinosaurs of the past. If scientists are successful in making monoclonal antibodies—and translating them into use on cancer patients, which is the current snag—the cancer drugs of the future will act like homing pigeons. Instead of blasting the entire body, cancer cells and normal cells alike, monoclonals will head directly to the cancer cells they are designed to treat. They will not harm a single, solitary normal cell.

Monoclonal antibodies are made like this: A mouse gets an injection of human cancer cells—the particular type of cancer that the doctor is trying to treat. Because this cancer is from a foreign body (at least as far as the mouse is concerned), the mouse has no trouble recognizing the antigen markers on the surface of the individual cancer cells. In response, the mouse's white blood cells—specifically, its B lymphocytes—begin to produce antibodies for the cancer cell antigens. These antibodies circulate through the bloodstream and hunt down the antigen markers for which they were created. When they locate them, they mark the cells the antigens are on—that is, the cancer cells—for destruction.

Next, some of the T lymphocyte cells that are producing these particular antibodies are extracted from the mouse. Then each one is chemically fused to a completely different cancer cell. This double cell is called a "hybridoma."

The hybridoma, made up of a cancer cell plus an antibody-producing white blood cell, has two important qualities, which you could say it has inherited from its two parents.

From the cancer side of the family, the new cell gets the characteristic of being able to divide forever. That's one of the qualities of cancer cells that were discussed in Chapter 1; cancer cells continue to divide regardless of whether there is a need for new cells.

From the white blood cell side of the family, the hybridoma inherits the ability to produce antibodies that can track down particular antigens—in this case the particular antigens found on the cells of the type of cancer the doctors are trying to treat, the one injected into the mouse in the first place.

In a laboratory dish, the hybridoma starts dividing, and never stops dividing. It makes exact copies, or clones, of itself, all of which contain the necessary antibody. Next, these antibodies are separated from the hybridomas.

Finally, the antibodies are injected into the bloodstream of the cancer patient and, according to the theory, off they go seeking *only* the cancer cells for which they were created. They ignore any other cells they meet up with along the way.

When they arrive at the cancer cells, they mark them for destruction. T lymphocyte white blood cells come in and finish the job.

So far, experiments with monoclonal antibodies have only been conducted on a small number of cancer patients. Most of them have been done on patients with leukemia or cancer of the lymphatic system. Since both of these types of cancer move throughout the body via one of its systems, it may be easier for monoclonal antibodies to spot the cancer cell antigens for which they were created.

In some research centers, scientists are experimenting with monoclonal antibodies in another way. They are adding other items to the antibody. In some cases, that item is a cancer-killing drug; in other cases, it is a radioactive material that allows the monoclonal antibody to be used as a diagnostic tool.

Imagine a cancer-killing drug attached to an antibody roaming around looking for its proper antigen mate, the cancer cell. Then zap! The antibody attaches itself to the cancer cell and releases its cancer-killing chemical.

As a diagnostic tool, monoclonal antibodies are fused with small amounts of radioactive material rather than cancer-killing drugs. The idea is to find tiny, secondary tumors that are too small to show up on an X-ray. Keep in mind that the earlier they are found, the easier these secondary tumors are to treat.

After the monoclonal antibodies have been fused to the radioactive material, the patient is placed under a scanning machine that is capable of picking up radiation. When these monoclonals are injected into the bloodstream, they head right for the cancer cells. Meanwhile, the machine follows the radiation in the cells. Within minutes, the scanner picks up the radiation which is, by then, at the cancer site, and the exact location of the tiny tumor is known.

Someday, these kinds of techniques may be available to

cancer patients around the world. Someday, more people will benefit from the research that is funded by the National Cancer Institute and the millions of dollars raised by cancer societies each year.

And yet, in spite of all these efforts, for many people who have cancer today these advances have not come fast enough. In desperation, many people turn to treatments that don't work. They are called "fringe methods" by researchers who work in the legitimate field of cancer treatment and research.

Fringe Methods

When you think about interferon and the premature hopes it created, you begin to see what can happen in the area of cancer treatment. An experiment that should be reported as preliminary research gets front-page billing. From it, readers infer that the cure for cancer is on the verge of being discovered. In certain newspapers that are more concerned about sales than facts, small bits of progress are even reported as THE CURE.

The legitimate therapies that now exist are unsuccessful for half the people who develop cancer. In a panic to do something, to do anything but give up, many people are tempted to seek out the promises that the proponents of the fringe methods make.

When all else has failed, when the proven treatments don't work anymore, some people will search frantically for anything that *might* help. For them, searching is better than doing nothing. While they are doing something, they can stop thinking about death.

But searching for fringe methods is a different story when a person who might have been cured by legitimate means delays seeking treatment. It is different when someone believes the illogical promises of an instant, complete cure. For this reason, it's important to understand why fringe methods don't work.

Every year, Americans spend between two and three *billion dollars* on potions, devices, and ceremonies that promise to cure cancer. Usually, these treatments also promise to accomplish the cure with no pain, and no suffering.

It's easy to see why people want to believe in them. Nonpoisonous injections can be pretty tempting to people who otherwise face chemotherapy. While coffee enemas may sound disgusting, they begin to sound a lot less terrible when the alternative is major surgery.

The best-known and most often tried method for fringe cancer therapy is laetrile. Its chemical name is amygdalin. It is also called vitamin B-17, cyto H-3, KH-3, and aprikern. Laetrile is found in apricot pits, peach pits, almonds, and apple seeds.

Those who support laetrile claim that it kills cancer cells when it releases cyanide, a deadly poison. In fact, laetrile does contain cyanide. That's part of the problem. Since cyanide is a deadly poison, it has been known to produce worse side effects than the proven anti-cancer chemicals.

Laetrile supporters insist that the cyanide stays locked in the laetrile except when it happens upon cancerous cells. They attribute this to the fact that cancer cells supposedly contain large amounts of a protein called beta-glucosidase, which releases the cyanide. Normal cells, they say, don't contain very much of this protein, and for this reason remain unharmed.

Laetrile supporters also insist that healthy cells are further protected from the cyanide because they contain rhodanase, which is supposed to convert cyanide into a harmless substance. Cancer cells supposedly don't contain rhodanase.

The trouble with all these explanations is that scientists have looked for beta-glucosidase in cancer cells and normal cells and have found only traces of it. As well, they have found no more, or less, of it in cancer cells than in normal cells. Scientists have also looked for rhodanase in both cancer cells and normal cells, and have found exactly the same amounts in both.

Nevertheless, because there has been so much controversy, and because so many people have been so interested in laetrile, many separate laetrile experiments have been conducted by scientists over the years. None have shown laetrile to be effective in the treatment of cancer.

And still the supporters of laetrile press on. Their claims are very similar to those of others who swear by drugs that scientists have proved useless. Some say that the medical community is plotting against them. Others insist that the medical community doesn't really want to see advances made in cancer research, because if cancer were cured, it would cost doctors their jobs.

There are other things that supporters of fringe therapies have in common with those who support laetrile. They all promote one type of treatment for all kinds of cancer. To them it makes no difference whatsoever that cancer is really a term for more than one hundred different diseases.

They tend not to publish the results of their studies, or the explanations of how these studies were conducted. Their records—if there are any records—are usually incomplete. When people insist that they have been miraculously cured of cancer, it is often discovered that no biopsies were ever performed. Whether or not the patient actually had cancer to begin with was frequently never proved.

Some people sell handwriting tests—one is called the Kanfer Neuromuscular—that are supposed to detect hidden cancers. Others sell grape cures. And there is the Orgone Energy Device, a gizmo which purports to harness energy from the universe to cure cancer.

Groups with highfalutin names like The Cancer Control Society, The Committee for Freedom of Choice in Cancer Therapy, and the National Health Federation support various fringe remedies. It's not so surprising that desperate people believe the stories that these organizations tell.

How Legitimate Research Works

Perhaps if people understood more about how legitimate scientists test cancer drugs, the fallacy of the fringe drugs would become more apparent.

In legitimate medical research, the first step in the identification of new chemicals is called screening. Every year, approximately 150,000 new chemicals are developed worldwide. Since it would be impossible to test them all on humans, they are first tested on mice. If a chemical is found to affect cancer tumor growth, it goes on to the next phase.

In this second step, the chemical is identified. Once this has been completed, it is then tested on other animals: monkeys and dogs.

If the chemical is still found to be safe, it goes on to be tested on humans—under tightly controlled conditions.

There are four stages to the human-testing phase. During the first stage, a drug is only given to a cancer patient whose disease has not responded to any other proven therapy. These patients are informed of the risks involved and the probability of success. Often it's not great. Much of the knowledge that is gained at this stage has to do with determining the proper dose, rather than curing people.

When a safe dose is found, the second phase begins. Studies are conducted to determine if the drug affects the growth rate of tumors in humans, and if so, which types of tumors respond.

In the following phases, these drugs are compared with others that are already in use. It is not until the fourth phase that a cancer drug actually makes it into the arsenal of drug therapies.

Since 1955, something like half a million drugs have been tested. Only one of every five thousand drugs even reaches the human testing phase. Fewer than one of every fifty thousand drugs tested has ended up on the cancer drug list. So far there are about forty, and only thirty are commonly used. It is an extensive and serious testing procedure.

But there is another truth to think about in the face of all this. Even after all the years of research, the time and money, the hopes and dreams, for more than half of the people who develop cancer, there is no long-term cure. *That* is the terrible truth.

One question remains: What do you do when there really is nothing left to think about but death?

CHAPTER FIVE
Dying with Cancer

I T CAN happen suddenly, like a brick shattering a pane of glass. You find out that someone you care about has cancer and that they are going to die.

Other times, the realization seeps into the consciousness slowly. Someone is in the middle of treatment and things begin to go badly. One day there is a vague feeling, perhaps because of a comment made by a doctor, or a bit of information in a pamphlet, that clicks. This treatment is not working, and it is not going to work. The doctors are doing all they can, but it is not enough. Perhaps it won't happen tomorrow, or next week, or even next month . . . but sometime soon this person will be a victim of cancer.

The way our society has looked at death, and the ways in which it has tried to cope with it, have changed slowly over the past thirty years.

In the 1950s, very few people would talk about death or dying. Most people bore the pain of watching a loved one die without any conversation about how they felt. Perhaps this had to do with the fact that the science of death and dying had not yet been created. I also suspect that people were embarrassed to admit that they sometimes felt angry as well as sad.

In the early 1960s, a few people, mostly psychiatrists, started talking and writing about death. A few years later, a handful of people in England began building homes, called "hospices," where people who were dying could live comfortably until the end came. Organizations were started to help people and their families who were trying to cope emotionally with dying and death.

In the 1980s, courses about death and dying were actually developed by professors in universities.

As a result of all this, many people are now trying to understand death as a natural part of the process of life—even when the person who is dying is not old.

Regarding death as natural doesn't mean that people handle it all that much better, or grieve any less. It just means that they believe that talking openly, instead of hiding their feelings, can help them to understand this aspect of life a little better. From a period of mourning, and a time of trying to make some sense out of something that is inexplicable, they hope to gather enough strength to be able to go on with their own lives, while at the same time cherishing the memory of the person who has died.

Why did people begin to change their attitude toward coping with death and dying? The question is difficult to answer.

One theory is that this new attitude evolved slowly because of natural events. In the 1960s, a few people came to the conclusion that they would be better able to cope with death if they didn't hide their feelings. They talked openly, wrote books about their experiences, built hospices, and eventually developed courses to teach others what they had discovered. As more people were exposed to the concept of examining their feelings, their experiences also changed. And as more people's experiences changed, new books were written and the original philosophy developed even more. These events were all intertwined. They were both the cause and the effect, and once they gained momentum, there was no way society could turn back.

Historians frequently ask themselves how events get started in the first place. Those who have chosen to investigate the issue of death and dying talk about how our society has changed from being largely rural to largely urban. Dr. Dorothy Ley, executive director of The Palliative Care Foundation of Canada, is one of these people.

"In the early part of this century," says Dr. Ley, "the

majority of people lived on farms rather than in cities. On farms, dying and death are more natural aspects of life." Dr. Ley is not trying to suggest that people who grew up on farms in the 1920s or 30s seeing farm animals die would have felt that the death of a relative was *easy* to accept. What she was suggesting was that because of their experiences, it may have seemed more logical to them that people do sometimes die before they are old.

Today, most people grow up in towns and cities; possibly you are one. It may be that you have never before had to think about death in any context. When people have no personal experience with a topic, they tend to turn to intellectual pursuits, like reading books, taking courses, or just talking to others. Some historians believe that this is what began to happen with the subject of death and dying as society became more urban.

When the "extended" family began to disappear—when mothers, fathers, grandparents, and perhaps even a few aunts or uncles no longer lived with all the children under one roof—this theme developed more. When there was no longer someone around to provide comfort in a time of crisis, people turned to society for assistance more frequently, and the concept of hospices and palliative care emerged. Perhaps, as people began to believe that society would take care of their needs, they began to feel more relaxed about moving far away from their families.

Within a generation or two of all these changes, another important development took place. Around the early 1950s, doctors and their patients began to believe that almost all sickness could be cured. New machines and new drugs—such as penicillin and the antibiotics that are now commonplace—were turning the practice of medicine into the most exciting science on earth. When people started to see pneumonia patients, for example, being cured for the first time, it gave them another reason to stop accepting death as normal.

Medical students in the 1960s didn't have time to think about death and dying; they had enough trouble keeping up with all the advances in medicine that were being developed to keep people alive.

Doctors who could suddenly cure people—of polio, of pneumonia, of influenza—didn't want to dwell on those who were dying. To some doctors, a dying patient meant failure, and many did not want to be reminded that it was still possible to fail.

A lot of emotional problems followed in the wake of all these changes, and today, many people are searching for a balance. Doctors are still trying to learn better methods of treatment. But they are now also trying to remember that people who are dying, and their families, must cope with how they feel.

The science of caring for people who are dying, called "palliative care," began with a few courageous pioneers.

In England in the 1960s, a physician who was knighted for her efforts, Dame Cicely Saunders, raised some money and built a home. She called it St. Christopher's. It was the first hospice.

At St. Christopher's, people who were specially trained took care of men and women who *knew* they were going to die. It was the first "free-standing" building whose staff focused their efforts on palliative care.

The word "hospice" comes from a Greek word which means "a resting place during a difficult journey." The journey, in this case, is from life to death.

The philosophy of palliative care is to ensure that people are made as comfortable and as fulfilled as possible during this difficult journey. It is different from "curative care," for which the hope is always that patients can be cured, or at least have their lives extended for a reasonable length of time.

Places like St. Christopher's are not like ordinary hospitals. There are doctors and nurses who do tests and give drugs. But if someone needs a pain-killer—although fewer than half of all cancer patients suffer pain in the last weeks of their lives—the medical staff does everything it can to stop the pain. Instead of trying to cure people, staff members try to provide people with comfort.

If a patient needs someone to talk to, a hand to hold, or someone who simply understands the fear that can go along with knowing you are going to die, the hand, the talk, or the understanding will be there. At a hospice, this kind of comfort is available during the day, and in the dark, lonely hours of the night. As long as a person is alive, the objective is to make every hour as fine as is humanly possible.

Hospices have another goal as well. The philosophy is that when someone who is dying has a family, the members of that family are dying a little too. A son, daughter, wife, husband, mother, father, sister, brother—each person in that family has a need, and each need is recognized as different. There are no rules about visiting hours at places like St. Christopher's; dying is a family affair.

It shocked me when I first heard it put that way—a family affair. To me family affairs have always been weddings, birthdays, and all sorts of happy occasions that I don't normally associate with death. In my family, when someone was dying or had died, we were supposed to act sad. At the same time, we were supposed to pretend that we were strong. Most important, we were not supposed to admit that we felt all the different emotions that people usually feel when someone close to them has died.

Is that how it is at a hospice? Well, "yes and no," is what people who work at places like St. Christopher's would say. They would say yes, because we all feel sad when we must say good-bye forever to someone we love, and sometimes we do pretend that we're strong to make it easier for the dying person. But they would also say no, because saying good-bye means remembering some good times, and maybe some bad times, as well. It also sometimes means feeling angry or deserted, even though it's illogical to blame someone who is about to die. It's also sometimes hard to separate emotions like sadness, and anger, and relief.

At the same time as the first hospices were being built in England, Dr. Elisabeth Kubler-Ross, a psychiatrist, was beginning to talk and write about dying and death in the United States.

For the first time, people in North America were hearing that the emotions which they were feeling affected others as well. They were finally hearing that it was normal to feel what they thought were negative emotions such as anger and relief. Reading Dr. Kubler-Ross's words made them realize that they were not the only ones who felt this way and, perhaps more important, that they were not crazy.

To explain to others what happens when people find out that they are going to die, Dr. Kubler-Ross came up with the concept of five "stages of dying." She calls them denial, anger, bargaining, depression, and acceptance. I never got the impression that Dr. Kubler-Ross meant these five stages to be taken literally—first this happens, then that happens, and that's that. When I first read about the stages of dying, many years ago, I took them to be concepts. I saw them as a way of explaining some of the things I had always sensed, but never seen put into words.

Not everyone who is dying goes through Dr. Kubler-Ross's five stages. Some people do not go through any of these stages at all. Others go through them in a different order, or miss one or more stages completely.

I think it has been a tragic error that, in an attempt to make some sense out of something as complex as death, some people looked at what Dr. Kubler-Ross wrote and accepted it at face value. Instead of realizing that each person is unique, they interpreted her ideas as gospel. Some people believed that these five labels alone could be used to conquer emotional pain. The interpretation was far too simplistic.

Dr. Kubler-Ross calls the first stage of dying "denial." When people are told that their disease is "terminal," that it cannot be cured and they are going to die, they may say something like: "I don't believe it. It's not true. You read the tests wrong. They got my name wrong. Whatever the screw-up is, this is not happening to me." Many people who are told, or who find out, that they have terminal cancer are unable to face it, at least for a while.

Sometimes the members of the dying person's family are also unable to believe the truth. Dr. Kubler-Ross's stages are usually used to describe what people who are dying go through, but their families often go through the same, or similar, stages at the same time, or at a different time. A doctor explains that there is nothing more to be done, and yet, it doesn't register. Families pretend that the type of treatment being given is still curative, rather than palliative.

Kassy is one of the many teenagers I spoke to about death and dying. She is sixteen now. When she was fourteen, her father, Michael, was diagnosed as having inoperable lung cancer. By the time it was discovered, the disease was so advanced that no curative treatment was feasible. Michael was sent home, where he remained for three months. Shortly after Kassy's fifteenth birthday, Michael returned to hospital, where he died after several weeks. A year has passed since then.

"I was away when my father found out he had lung cancer and only a few months to live," Kassy told me. "I was visiting my friend Cathy for the summer. Her parents didn't tell me about Daddy. He wouldn't let them. He wanted to wait until I came home so he could tell me himself. When he told me he was dying, it was as if a special part of him trusted me enough to say it. 'I won't have you for very much longer, Kassy,' he said.

"We both cried. We held onto each other, and as long as my arms were around him, I was sure everything would be okay. I didn't believe it. He was just very sick. He'd get better, I knew that he would."

Kassy's mother, Florence, had been with Michael when the doctor had told him the results of the biopsy. It had revealed a large cancerous tumor in Michael's left lung. That was in July, almost a month before Kassy came home.

Florence: "We didn't believe it at first either. I don't think most people do; it's too much of a shock. But I realize now that we made a mistake in waiting so long to bring Kassy home. We thought we could spare her some of the pain. Now I realize that what Michael and I went through those first few weeks, pretending it wasn't true, is what Kassy had to go through alone in August. Maybe it would have been better for all of us to have done it together at once, but how do you know at the time?"

Kassy: "Everyone has to choose their own way of handling things. I would never tell anyone to do it my way. It was just what I needed to do. For me, my dad's dying was like a play, and I picked my part and played it as well as I could. I played the tough one, pretending it would all be over soon. He'd come home and life would get back to normal.

"He knew what I was up to. He'd tease me and say, 'Kassy, you can get mad in front of me. You can cry. I used to be mad about this too.' And I'd say to him, 'There's nothing to be mad about, Daddy. This will all be over soon.' I meant that the bad dream would be over, not that he'd die."

Dr. Kubler-Ross says that many of the people she has talked to refused to believe that they were dying, and that for some people this is a necessary and helpful stage. Denying the truth is one method people use to protect themselves from shock, until a traumatic concept has had a chance to mellow. Usually within a few days, or a few weeks, the truth does sink in.

For a few people, however, it is better never to face the truth. Some people die never having given up their belief that they are going to be cured. According to Dr. Kubler-Ross, however, this doesn't happen all that often. Most people first deny that they are going to die, and then get angry when they realize it is true. She calls this next stage "anger." Most of the time, the people who are close to someone who is dying also go through a period of feeling angry.

It can break your heart when you think of what frequently happens when someone who is dying gets angry. On the one hand, it makes perfect sense. When people realize that they are going to die, they also realize that they are going to lose all the people they love.

But on whom do they take out their anger? Usually, it's on the people they care about most, or on the nurses who are trying to make them comfortable. When family members don't understand what is happening—or when they do but can't take it anymore—some of them try to find excuses for staying away. When they stay away, the person who is dying gets even more angry. "I am dying, and they don't even care."

Florence: "Michael was like that most of July. He was impossible. It's horrible to say, but he drove me up a wall. I wanted to be with him so much, to spend those last few months talking about the good times we'd had. Some days I'd try to talk to him and he'd shout at me to get out of the room. I didn't understand that it meant he finally knew he was going to die. In one way I'm glad Kassy never saw any of this. She was his special one, and she idolized him."

Kassy: "By September, even I knew it was true. That was when I began to ask myself what kind of lousy God would take a man like my dad. Fifty-nine years old, just starting to think about retiring, and having some time to spend with my mom. At night I'd beat up my teddy bear, smash him against the wall. During the day I thought the doctors must be jerks; what did they mean there was *nothing* they could do? Then I'd hate myself for wanting to just hold him in my arms and cry forever. . . ."

Dr. Kubler-Ross went on to describe what often happens next. She calls it "bargaining." The patient who is dying may say something like, "Okay, I get the picture, but please"—often the please is directed at God—"don't let me die until my son's wedding; until my daughter's baby is born; until the crocuses bloom in the spring."

It is a time of hope, of false dreams, and of families not knowing how to react. Should they go along with the bargains, or try to explain that they really don't make too much sense? Or are they making some bargains of their own, knowing all along that they are doing exactly that?

And is honesty always best, anyway? Would it necessarily be any better if no bargains were made? No one knows the answers to these questions, not even Dr. Elisabeth Kubler-Ross.

Kassy: "I promised myself that I'd never get angry again, that I'd be strong for him. If I could be strong, then he'd be okay. If I was weak, he'd die. But he'd say, 'Kassy, you can cry. I know you want to cry.' And I'd tell him, 'Oh no, I don't.'

"By then, in September, I think he was way beyond any

point I ever got to until almost a year later. By then, dying made some sort of weird sense to him. He tried to explain it to me once, but I couldn't understand."

Most professionals agree that families who try to talk about these questions—even when they have no answers—are able to cope with death a little better than families where what's happening is not talked about at all. Still, while it's true that today more families are able to discuss death and dying than thirty years ago, not many are very good at it. Most people are still brought up to keep their grief to themselves.

"Depression" is the name Dr. Kubler-Ross gives to the fourth stage of dying. It is the time for grief, for tears, and for despair. Psychiatrists and psychologists agree that while a dying person, or a relative, is depressed, it is not the time to try and cheer them up. It is the time to be silent, to hold someone's hand, or to share someone's tears.

Kassy: "When school started, everything seemed to change for me. I got so moody. I couldn't concentrate. I'd be sitting in class and the teacher would call my name and it would take me a minute before I even knew what class I was in. Some of my teachers understood and stayed off my back, but a few of them made me feel like a fool in front of the whole class. They'd catch me staring out the window, or reading the wrong page."

Florence: "She was so quiet about it then, so sad those last couple of months before Michael died. I think it was easier for Barbara, Kassy's older sister. She could let herself fall apart; she spent most of those last months crying. Kassy would try to comfort her.

"For a while there, Kassy and I changed roles. She became the mother and I became the little girl, if that makes any sense. I guess I was more like Barbara than Kassy. I'd ask what to wear, what to cook. For a long time, after Michael died, it was difficult for Kassy to go back to being the youngest child. I think Barbara and I went through a lot of our grieving while Michael was dying. . . . Kassy didn't even start grieving until he had been dead for several months."

You hear about people who are dying reaching the stage

Dr. Kubler-Ross calls "acceptance." They feel at peace with themselves and with the world. Sometimes members of their families are able to accept it too, other times not. I don't think, however, that people accept death quite as often as professionals would like to believe. One thing that has always bothered me about the idea of acceptance is the unspoken implication that the dying person who *doesn't* find peace has failed, and that the family has somehow failed too. This happens frequently when someone is dying of cancer.

Kassy: "I know that they all felt better about it than I did at the end. I just kept feeling worse and worse, and feeling guilty about that. Those last few weeks, I couldn't stand seeing him. I went to the hospital less and less. I couldn't bear to see him slowly turning into someone I didn't know. I couldn't stand the way he would sometimes smile at me through the pain and the drugs they kept shooting into him. One day I'd be so mad. The next day I would be back to not believing it was true. The day after that I'd just lock myself in my room and cry."

Cancer patients, and their families, often know for a number of months, sometimes for years, that death is inevitable. When the process of dying goes on for so long, people sometimes go through Dr. Kubler-Ross's stages forward, or backward, and often more than once. Which stage, if any, a person happens to be in at the time of death depends on many, many things.

The same stages sometimes start all over again for the family members after the person has died.

Kassy: "For six months I couldn't believe he was dead. It was as if he were just on another one of his business trips, coming home in two weeks. I'd hear a car pull into the driveway and I'd say to Barbara, 'Daddy's home.' When reality finally settled in, it was her turn to comfort me.

"I think part of me tried to keep busy so I'd have no time to think about the truth: he was dead. It's hard to explain because you'd think I would have wanted some time to myself to be able to see things clearly. But I preferred life to be a jumble.

"I'd offer to cook dinner. I'd bake chocolate chip cookies for Barbara. I remember one time she asked me why I never made chocolate cake. I went crazy; I told her to take the cookies and do you know what with them. I thought 'Dammit, get off my back. I'm only fifteen, just leave me the hell alone.' And yet I had been the one to offer. I was the one who always wanted to keep busy, because when they did leave me alone it was worse. When I had time on my hands I could think clearly, and I had to face the truth. It wasn't a play; he wasn't coming home. Then I'd go back to being busy all the time, and my little fantasy would continue."

Florence: "I didn't know what to do with her. My heart would break. Why couldn't she accept it, at least realize that it was true? It made Barbara and me feel guilty. We had loved Michael too, but we knew it was time to get on with our own lives."

Kassy: "It's taken me almost a year to get myself together. I'm getting back to my schoolwork a little more now. I think about him a little less—twice a day, instead of twice an hour. A month ago, I took his picture out of the drawer where I had put it the day he died. It took that long before I could get used to the idea of looking at him every day. I've never told this to anyone before, but the day he died, I felt like throwing that photograph against the wall. It must be hard to understand why anyone would want to do that to someone they love so much, but I did. When he first died, I hated him for leaving me, as if it had been his fault."

Florence: "Having someone you love die that way changes you forever. Part of you feels that you'll never be whole again, never know an hour of peace. Another part loses some of the ability to feel pain. Little things that used to be such a big deal to me don't seem so important anymore. I don't know if that contradiction makes any sense."

Kassy: "I carry a sadness in my heart. I wear it like someone else would wear a bracelet or a ring. Things strike me from a weird angle. To most people, butter pecan ice cream on a fall afternoon is just a treat. To me, it's what

Daddy was trying to eat one day the last week, biting off the bottom of the cone like a kid, sucking the butter pecan ice cream through as if it were a straw.

"Sometimes I read over the poems I've written and I wonder about loving and hating and how they can seem the same. But I know other kids who've had a mother or father die of cancer and some of them say they know what I mean. It helps, you know, to find out that you're not the only weirdo who can't stand how she feels."

In North America, many of the people who die of cancer die in regular hospitals, sometimes in a palliative care ward but more often in a regular ward that is dedicated to curative care. The rest die at home, either with or without some amount of support from professionals who have training in palliative care. There are approximately 1,400 palliative care operations on the entire North American continent. Some of them are free-standing hospices. More are contained within hospitals. Still others are run on a home-care basis, but it is rare for home-care services to be provided on other than a drop-in basis. It has been estimated that, of the half a million people in North America who die of cancer each year, only about 100,000 receive any palliative care at all.

Some people, like Dr. Ley, argue further that palliative care does not work properly in a hospital setting, that a home-like atmosphere cannot be duplicated in a hospital—even a separate wing of a hospital—whose main focus is curative care. Dr. Ley, and the people who support her efforts, want to see more and better home-care support programs. They believe that many cancer patients could remain at home to die if their families could rely on the kind of community support that is commonplace in England where the palliative care philosophy began.

Florence: "We didn't know what to do. Michael wanted so badly to stay at home for the end, to die in his own house. Our medical insurance included home care, but this only meant that a nurse would come by to give him his shots. We didn't have the money for nursing care twenty-four hours a day, and that's what he needed near the end."

I have talked to many people who wish, with all their hearts, that they had time to think about emotions and the stages of dying. But there is so little time when there are so many practical decisions to be made.

Should someone who is dying remain at home? Many hospital settings aren't exactly personal, but if a person who is dying does come home, how does the family cope? It seems horrible to be thinking about details like who will cook and who will clean when someone is dying. But these details have to be considered. Someone has to think about them.

Kassy: "For me it was like therapy. I cooked and cleaned to keep from facing the truth. Someone I know, a friend whose mother was dying of breast cancer, resented having to do all the chores. All she ever talked about was 'getting the hell away.' "

Some families do try and keep the person who is dying at home. When they can get a bit of help from a day nurse, or a housekeeper, it often works pretty well. But many families I have spoken to have had to send the dying person back to the hospital near the end. Caring for someone twenty-four hours a day is sometimes too much for a family to bear.

Florence: "We couldn't have done it for those last three weeks. It's as simple as that. I can remember a few friends saying, 'You're going to let him stay home, aren't you?' What a fantasy!"

People who are dying of cancer have special needs, as the cancer cells begin to monopolize the nutrition that normal cells need. Cancer patients require special diets. Often they don't feel like eating, or can't keep many types of food down. Sometimes they need pain-killers which can only be given by injection. Other times they need help to just eat, or go to the bathroom—all the things we normally don't think about twice.

The saddest part, I think, is the guilt people sometimes

feel about not being able to cope. Guilt is a word that came up often when I was speaking to people who loved someone who was dying of cancer.

Florence: "At first I did feel guilty. I knew staying at home was what Michael really wanted. But people who aren't in the middle of all this don't understand. It's easy for them to say *everyone* should be able to die at home."

I spoke to people who were dying of cancer and felt guilty for being so helpless. I spoke to people who were trying to help them, and they felt guilty about not helping enough.

My impression was that teenagers often feel the most guilt of all. Those are the years when it is time to explore the world, to feel proud of newly found independence, to break loose. At the same time, it is the age to begin to share part of the burden. One day they want to, the next day they don't.

The pages you have just been reading took a year to write. Should I even include a section on death and dying in this book, I kept asking myself. Once I decided that I was right to have done it, I started to wonder if I should have mentioned concepts like palliative care or people like Dr. Elisabeth Kubler-Ross.

"What if . . . ?" I kept asking this same question of every doctor and social worker I talked to about this part of the book: "What if people trying to cope with someone who has cancer read about all the problems other people are having—with guilt and anger—and they're not having any problems at all? What if they read what I write and end up thinking there's something wrong with them for feeling okay? What if they end up, *because of what I write*, experiencing guilt?"

I worried about this for weeks. And then the weeks became months and I started dreaming about it. It got to the point where I was so worried that I wrote nothing. I couldn't finish this book.

It went on until one day I met Dr. Stephen Fleming, a psychology professor at Toronto's York University.

"I'm not getting anywhere," I told him. "I'm doing nothing but worrying about causing people a lot of grief."

Dr. Fleming smiled as he told me very simply, "Of all the things you have to worry about, you don't have to worry about that!

"A few people," he continued, "a very few people will go through the experience of someone they care about dying of cancer and get through it without too much grief.

"They'll read what other people have to say and feel lucky. The rest, you know, all go through the same things. It can only help them to find out that there are others who are feeling the same way."

I thought about it and began to realize that what Dr. Fleming was saying made sense. The fifty people I had talked to over an eighteen-month period had indeed had very similar things to say about what it's like to love someone who is dying or someone who has died already. I began to realize that there had been times during those months when I could have finished any sentence that someone had begun.

"You won't believe it," someone would start out, and because I had heard it before, I knew by the tone in the forlorn voice that I was about to hear once again how guilty someone felt for being angry. "I got so mad at him for getting sick. How can you be angry at someone with cancer who is going to die?"

But I heard it more times than I can count. The teenagers especially shared so many feelings. I wished at times that they all could have met to trade stories. That way, they would have known for sure that almost everyone feels neglected and overprotected at the same time.

I thought about one high school student in particular who felt neglected one week and utterly nagged the next. "How can it be that one minute my parents act as if they couldn't care less about what I do and the next minute they're breathing down my neck?"

It was a good question—how can it be?

I asked a few of their parents. "Your kids say you're driving them nuts. They talk about the hard times they are having. Can you see it? Are you acting a bit weird?"

Mostly I got gestures rather than answers. Hands thrown up in the air, sighs, and tear-filled eyes that looked as if they wanted to drift off into space rather than face the answers to those questions.

"How can I tell my daughter that I'm coming apart at the seams?" a man whose wife was dying of stomach cancer asked me. "She needs me to be strong, and I feel as if I'm six years old. Are you crazy? Of course I'm acting weird."

In the 1960s, doctors like Elisabeth Kubler-Ross made up labels like "bargaining" and "denial," but ordinary people have been *living* these labels for many, many years. Mothers have been acting like their young daughters, fathers like their sons. But what may be worse for parents is that they probably feel doubly guilty when they cannot be strong. Parents wish they knew what to do, what to say, and how to protect their children from the worst. With the best of intentions, they sometimes don't give them what they need.

And the point of saying all this? The point was made by another physician I spoke to, Dr. Saul Levine, chief of psychiatry at Toronto's Sunnybrook Hospital.

"Saul," I said to him just before leaving his office, "tell me, is hearing all this stuff really going to help these people?"

He thought for a few seconds before he answered: "Every time I have been faced with looking at who is the most helpful person in a crisis, any kind of crisis, I have usually found that it's other people who are going through the same thing, or have gone through it before.

"Everyone seems to have the same feeling: 'God, if I tell people how I feel, they'll think I'm off my rocker.' I hear this all the time. But, if people hear from someone else in the same boat what they themselves are thinking, they believe that they're not alone. It's different, often much better, than hearing it from a doctor. You find out that it's normal to feel whatever you do feel. It's a wonderful thing to discover that you're not nuts, or alone."

Perhaps your own situation is completely different from Kassy's, but you *feel* the same way. Or maybe the scene is the same, but the players are different. Never mind. The point is, I think, the very one Dr. Levine repeated as I left. "When someone you love is dying of cancer, *whatever* you feel is normal."

Somewhere—I guarantee it—someone else knows exactly what you're going through.

PART II
The Common Cancers

The Carcinomas

Carcinomas are cancers that begin in epithelial cells. These are the cells that line the inside and outside surfaces of the body's organs.

Skin Cancer

What is the skin?
The skin is a huge organ that protects the body from injury, excretes waste products, and regulates body temperature.

What is skin cancer?
Like other carcinomas, skin cancer develops in the epithelial cells that form the lining of the skin. There are three main types of epithelial skin cells: basal cells, squamous cells, and melanoma cells. Skin cancer can start to grow in any of these three types of skin cells.

Who gets skin cancer and what is the outlook?
Skin cancer is the most common type of cancer; in North America, approximately 439,000 new cases are diagnosed each year. About 95 percent of them begin in either squamous or basal cells, and because they are slow-growing and

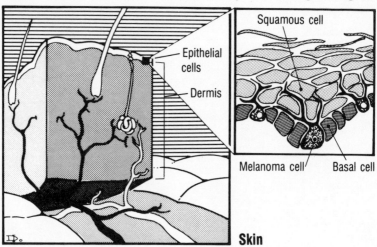

Epithelial cells

Dermis

Squamous cell

Melanoma cell   Basal cell

Skin

tend not to spread, are completely curable almost 100 percent of the time.

Malignant melanoma, the one type of skin cancer that is difficult to treat, grows and spreads quickly. Fortunately it is rare, and can be cured when it is detected at an early stage. Malignant melanoma is diagnosed in approximately 23,000 North Americans each year, almost two-thirds of whom can be cured.

What causes skin cancer and who is at high risk?

Skin cancer is most often caused by long-term overexposure to the ultraviolet rays of the sun, although some chemical pollutants can cause it as well. For this reason, cancer of the skin tends to show up on areas of the body—the face, the backs of the hands—that are exposed to the environment. Because these areas are also visible, skin cancer rarely remains undetected for very long.

Dark-skinned people—whose skin cells contain large amounts of melanin, which filters out ultraviolet rays—are less susceptible to skin cancer than light-skinned people.

Farmers, fishermen, and sailors, who work in the sun, as well as avid sunbathers, also tend to develop skin cancer more frequently than other people.

The signs and symptoms of skin cancer

The easier-to-cure types of skin cancer usually show up as pale, wax-like, pearly nodules or red, scaly patches.

Malignant melanoma usually starts out as a small, mole-like growth which then begins to get bigger, and changes color or shape. Sometimes a malignant melanoma will itch.

The diagnosis of skin cancer

Suspicious-looking skin conditions are biopsied incisionally if they are large, and excisionally if they are small. This minor surgical procedure can usually be performed in a doctor's office with only a local anesthetic. The biopsy is then sent to a lab to be examined for cancerous cells.

The treatment of skin cancer

Surgery, radiation, electrodesiccation, and cryosurgery are

used to treat the two common types of skin cancer. Electrodesiccation destroys tissues by using heat. Cryosurgery destroys tissue by freezing it.

Surgery is the most common treatment for malignant melanoma, although radiation therapy or chemotherapy is sometimes used when it has spread.

Lung Cancer

What are the lungs?
The lungs are a pair of elastic organs that are used for breathing.

What is lung cancer?
Lung cancer is a type of carcinoma that generally develops in the epithelial cells that form the interior lining of the airways to the lungs. This is because the airways get the most exposure to inhaled pollutants; almost everyone who develops this type of lung cancer smokes. A rarer type of lung cancer can begin in the epithelial cells of the "outlying" regions of a lung; non-smokers sometimes develop this type of lung cancer.

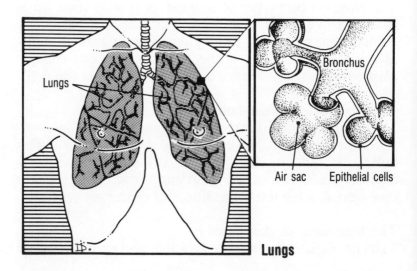

Lungs

Who gets lung cancer and what is the outlook?
Lung cancer kills more North Americans than any other kind of cancer. During 1985, approximately 155,000 North Americans learned that they had lung cancer, and about 136,000 died of this disease. These numbers have been increasing, especially among females. Lung cancer is the leading cause of death from cancer in males, and researchers are predicting that it will surpass breast cancer to become the leading cause of death from cancer in females within a couple of years.

The overall prognosis—a medical term that describes what will probably happen to one person, given what has already happened to others in the same situation—for lung cancer is bleak. More than 90 percent of lung cancer patients die within five years.

If a former lung cancer patient is alive and symptom-free five years after treatment, it is unlikely that cancerous lung cells will reappear; these rare individuals are considered to be cured.

What causes lung cancer and who is at high risk?
Smoking is the main cause of lung cancer. The more and the longer a person smokes, the greater his or her risk of developing lung cancer. More than 90 percent of lung cancer patients are smokers.

People who have smoked a pack or more of cigarettes a day for many years—perhaps as many as twenty—have the greatest risk of developing lung cancer. According to some studies, a person who starts smoking at age fifteen is thirty times more likely to develop lung cancer by age thirty-five than someone who has never smoked.

People who are exposed to asbestos, chromium, nickel, coal tars, or radioactive uranium—usually because of their jobs—also have a higher-than-average risk of developing lung cancer. Non-smokers are less affected by these substances than smokers.

Lung cancer can be prevented. The best protection is never to start smoking. The next-best protection is to quit if you already smoke. When a person stops smoking, his or her risk of developing lung cancer stops increasing. Ten to fifteen years after quitting, a former smoker—even a former long-term, heavy smoker—has almost the same risk of developing lung cancer as a person who has never smoked.

Inhaling smoke and other pollutants year after year damages the cleaning mechanism of the lungs. When the lungs can no longer clean themselves properly, inhaled carcinogenic substances build up and may eventually cause a growth gene to mutate. Some people smoke for years, however, and never develop lung cancer. It may be that their lungs are better than other people's at resisting the effects of these carcinogenic substances.

The signs and symptoms of lung cancer

Lung cancer is usually suspected when someone coughs up blood or complains of a hacking cough that continues to get worse; this is caused by the lungs trying to get rid of the foreign object—the tumor—that is lodged in an airway. If the tumor is large enough it can obstruct the passageway almost completely, and the patient will also experience chest pain and difficulty breathing.

The diagnosis of lung cancer

When symptoms such as these persist, an X-ray of the lungs is taken to determine if there is a tumor and where it is located. Usually some sputum—the technical term for spit—is examined for any cancer cells that the tumor may have shed. Often the doctor will examine the airway with a bronchoscope, a type of endoscope that can be inserted into the airway via the mouth. With a bronchoscope, the doctor can examine the airway for a tumor and, if there is one, take a biopsy of it. This biopsy will be sent to a lab for microscopic examination.

If the tumor is too far along a bronchial tube to be reached with a bronchoscope, it is more difficult to take a biopsy. In such a case, a fine needle must be inserted through the chest wall, using a special type of X-ray for guidance.

If the doctor suspects that nearby lymph nodes have trapped some cells shed by the tumor, a minor surgical procedure will be performed. A tube will be passed through a tiny slit above the breastbone, and a biopsy of a lymph node will be taken and examined in a lab.

If these lymph nodes contain cancer cells, it is likely that other tests will be performed to determine if the cancer has spread to more distant organs, and to what extent.

The treatment of lung cancer

There are many decisions to be made once a diagnosis of lung cancer is confirmed. Some types of lung cancer grow and spread very quickly; others grow relatively slowly and tend not to spread for a long time.

Surgery, radiation therapy, or chemotherapy, and sometimes a combination of the three, can be used to treat lung cancer.

If the tumor is localized to one particular spot, it can often be removed surgically. Unfortunately, only about one in five lung cancer patients is diagnosed when the tumor is still localized; of these, fewer than one in four is still alive five years after the initial diagnosis was made.

If the patient has other problems that preclude surgery, or if the tumor is not in an easy-to-reach place, radiation therapy is sometimes used.

If there is evidence that the tumor has spread to distant parts of the body, chemotherapy is sometimes used. Over the past few years there have been some good results using chemotherapy on patients with certain types of lung cancer.

In many cases, lung cancer is detected at such an advanced stage that only palliative care is feasible.

Breast Cancer

What is the breast?

The breast is a gland designed to secrete milk. It remains small in males, enlarges in females during adolescence, and enlarges further during pregnancy and when milk is produced. People tend to think of a breast as a single gland, but in fact each breast consists of between fifteen and twenty lobes, or segments. Each segment has a duct, and each duct opens onto the nipple.

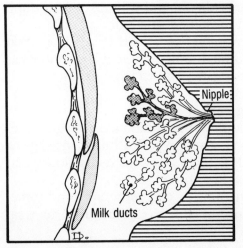

Breast

What is breast cancer?
Most breast cancers begin in the epithelial cells that line the milk ducts and milk sacs. Some breast cancers grow into the duct canal; others grow into the breast tissue itself.

Who gets breast cancer and what is the outlook?
Every year, approximately 134,000 North American women develop breast cancer, and approximately 42,000 women die of this disease. One in every 12 North American women will develop breast cancer at some point during her life. The disease is rare in women who are under the age of thirty, and becomes more common after the age of forty. Occasionally breast cancer develops in males, although it is usually detected early on and successfully treated.

Breast cancer in females can also be treated successfully in many cases. If it is detected when it is still localized, it can be cured 85 percent of the time.

Once breast cancer has spread to the nearby lymph nodes (at which point it is referred to as invasive breast cancer with regional involvement), the chances of a cure fall to slightly higher than 50 percent.

For breast cancer that is advanced when it is diagnosed, the outlook is usually grim.

While more North American women are developing

breast cancer than in the past, about the same number are dying of this disease each year. This means that treatment is successful in more cases.

When approximately sixteen years have passed, a former breast cancer patient is considered cured.

What causes breast cancer and who is at high risk?
Although scientists do not know the exact cause of breast cancer, diets that are high in fat are thought to increase a person's risk of developing this type of carcinoma. In countries like Japan, where people's diets are low in fat, the incidence of breast cancer is also low. In North America, the diet is generally high in fat and the incidence of breast cancer is also high.

The female sex hormone estrogen—which is contained in birth control pills—has been linked to breast cancer in animals. There is, however, no general link between the pill and breast cancer in humans. Women who are interested in taking birth control pills are advised to discuss the advantages and disadvantages of this method of birth control with a doctor, and to take as low a dose as possible.

Certain women seem to be more prone to breast cancer than other women.

A woman who has had breast cancer once has a greater chance of developing it again than a woman who has never had the disease. The higher risk may be caused by environmental factors, such as diet, that do not change.

A woman with more than one close relative who has had breast cancer—a mother and a sister, for example—has a higher risk of developing this disease than a woman whose family has no history of breast cancer. Researchers are not certain whether this is due to hereditary or environmental factors, but many researchers lean toward blaming the environment.

Women who have had a first child before the age of twenty-five seem to develop breast cancer less often than women who bear their first child after the age of thirty, or women who bear no children at all. Researchers do not understand why this is so.

Women who begin menstruating before the age of eleven,

or continue to menstruate after the age of fifty, also tend to have a higher-than-normal risk of developing breast cancer.

Some studies indicate that overweight, post-menopausal women develop breast cancer more frequently than women whose weight is normal.

Other studies show that women who have a history of non-malignant, or benign, breast tumors also have a higher-than-average risk of developing cancerous breast tumors.

The signs and symptoms of breast cancer
When a woman has breast cancer, there are usually no obvious symptoms, such as pain. When a tumor grows into a duct, however, there may be discharge or bleeding from a nipple.

Breast cancer surveillance
There are several ways of detecting breast cancer at an early stage. The easiest is through breast self-examination, which is usually called BSE. All women should practice BSE, but women over the age of thirty-five who are in a high-risk group should also discuss the various other available surveillance tests for breast cancer with a doctor. These tests include mammography and ultrasonography. Researchers are also working on a diagnostic blood test for breast cancer, and it is hoped that this simple type of test will be available to the public within a few years.

Studies have shown that women who practice BSE properly can detect early breast tumors that are no larger than the size of a pea. Women who discover breast tumors "by accident" often find tumors the size of a golf ball. The American and Canadian Cancer Societies distribute free pamphlets that show women how to do BSE. It is completely painless and takes no more than a couple of minutes each month. Many women also ask their doctor to examine their breasts and to make sure that they themselves are doing BSE properly.

A low-radiation-level X-ray called a mammogram is also used to detect early breast cancers in women who have stopped menstruating. For a number of years this type of

X-ray was used on premenopausal women as well. The studies that were done to evaluate mammography on premenopausal women, however, showed that it wasn't particularly helpful, and better methods of mammography are now being investigated by the American Breast Cancer Awareness Program and the Canadian National Breast-Screening Study.

In some research centers, ultrasound waves, which can detect breast tumors because they have a different density than normal breast tissue, are being used to detect breast cancer at an early stage.

The diagnosis of breast cancer
Any lump in a breast should be examined by a doctor immediately. If the lump appears to be a cyst—a sac filled with liquid—the area around the cyst can be frozen with a local anesthetic, and the fluid removed with a thin needle.

This fluid is sent to a lab and, if its cells are benign, which they are more than nine times out of ten, no further treatment is necessary.

Solid masses, however, must be biopsied.

Sometimes a biopsy can be taken in the doctor's office. The area is frozen with a local anesthetic, a tiny incision is made, and a piece of tissue is removed. Other times, a needle aspiration can be performed; a bit of tissue is sucked up with a thin needle.

In most cases, however, a general anesthetic and a surgical procedure are necessary. Often, the biopsy is sent to the lab while the patient remains under general anesthetic. This is done so that, if further surgery is required, the patient will not have to undergo a general anesthetic twice. More than eight out of ten solid tumors turn out to be benign.

The treatment of breast cancer
Surgery, radiation therapy, and chemotherapy—and frequently a combination of all three—are used to treat cancerous breast tumors.

While surgery is still the most common treatment, the disfiguring radical mastectomy is no longer frequently performed. Instead of resecting the cancerous tumor along with the entire breast, all the lymph nodes in the area of the breast, and the muscle beneath the breast—for that is what radical breast surgery involves—other types of surgery remove much less.

The least radical type of breast surgery is lumpectomy. The tumor, a margin of normal breast tissue as a preventive measure, and usually a number of nearby lymph nodes are resected. The lymph nodes are examined in a lab for cancerous cells.

An important 1985 study compared the results of mastectomy and lumpectomy on women who had breast tumors that measured no more than four centimeters in diameter when they were first detected. The research involved 1,843 patients: about a third were treated with mastectomy, a third with lumpectomy, and the rest with a combination of lumpectomy and radiation. (Those women whose lymph nodes were also found to be cancerous were given adjuvant chemotherapy as well.) The results of the study showed that there was no advantage to having a mastectomy rather than a lumpectomy. In fact, the women who had the highest rate of success were those who had a lumpectomy plus radiation treatment.

Sometimes, the entire breast is removed—a simple mastectomy—and perhaps some lymph nodes, but nothing else.

Other times, the breast, some tissue of the armpit, and perhaps some lymph nodes—but not the muscle—are removed. This procedure is called a modified radical mastectomy.

When radiation therapy is used, the tumor is exposed to destructive cobalt rays.

If cancer cells from a breast tumor have already metastasized from the primary tumor, chemotherapy is frequently used.

Adjuvant chemotherapy is now also frequently used immediately following surgery or radiation therapy, *before* there is any sign of a secondary tumor. The aim of adjuvant chemotherapy is to kill any shed cells before they have a chance to grow into a tumor. The results of the initial studies on adjuvant chemotherapy are not yet complete, but some doctors feel that better cure rates for breast cancer are going to show up with this type of chemotherapy.

Hormone therapy is also sometimes used for certain types of breast cancer that depend upon a particular hormonal environment in order to grow.

Sometimes, if the hormonal balance can be changed by either adding or subtracting hormones, a cancerous breast tumor will shrink, instead of growing.

To reduce the amount of a particular hormone, the organ that produces the hormone is removed surgically, or destroyed by radiation. The ovaries, for example, produce estrogen and are sometimes resected or destroyed by radiation. Drugs can also be given to inhibit the production of certain hormones.

If more of a certain hormone is required, it can be given by pills or injections.

After the treatment
Many former breast cancer patients have emotional problems to face.

Although most women who have had a breast removed can return to their normal activities within a few weeks, some find that the fear of what life will be like with only one breast is overwhelming. A common worry is that the man in her life will no longer find her attractive. Or, if single, a woman may worry about being able to begin a relationship with a new man.

Some relationships do break up because of breast cancer, although most do not. And women who have had mastectomies do find they can begin new relationships.

Both the American and Canadian Cancer Societies have created a nationwide support service, called the Mastectomy Visiting Program, for women who have recently undergone treatment for breast cancer. Many women find it helpful to talk to someone who has shared the same experience. Other women want information about artificial breast forms, or about exercises that can help them cope better with the recovery process.

Reconstructive surgery to replace a missing breast, called mammoplasty, is becoming more and more common. In the past, some doctors scoffed at women who were concerned about replacing a lost breast. Today, most doctors acknowledge that, for some women, mammoplasty is beneficial and even necessary.

Prostate Cancer

What is the prostate?
The prostate is a gland that is part of the male reproductive system. It produces secretions that are important in the make-up of the semen.

What is prostate cancer?
Prostate cancer is a slow-growing cancer that generally begins to develop in the epithelial cells of the lining of the back of the prostate gland.

Who gets prostate cancer and what is the outlook?
The number of North American men who develop cancer of the prostate gland is second only to the number who develop lung cancer. Unlike lung cancer, prostate cancer can often be treated successfully. Of the approximately

Prostate

92,000 North American men who develop prostate cancer each year, about 70 percent can be treated successfully.

One of the reasons why so many prostate cancer patients survive is that it is one of the slowest growing of all cancers, and most prostate cancer patients are over the age of sixty-five when a tumor is first detected. In fact, the disease is sometimes discovered only when a person dies of something totally unrelated, and an autopsy reveals the presence of a cancerous prostate tumor.

Often, however, prostate cancer can be life-threatening. After a number of years, cells from a prostate cancer tumor usually spread into the lymph nodes nearby, or to other parts of the body via the bloodstream.

What causes prostate cancer and who is at high risk?
The causes and risk factors for prostate cancer are unknown.

The signs and symptoms of prostate cancer
Cancerous prostate tumors often cause no signs or symptoms at all. When there are symptoms, they are usually much the same as those associated with a more common, but benign, prostate problem in which the organ becomes swollen. They include: difficulty in urinating, frequent urination, blood in the urine, continuing low back pain, or pain in the pelvis or upper thighs.

The diagnosis of prostate cancer
When prostate cancer is suspected, the doctor will examine the area digitally—that is, with a finger—through the rectum. If a tumor is felt, minor surgery will be performed to take a biopsy, which usually requires only a brief hospital stay. If the biopsy reveals cancerous cells, it is likely that more tests will be performed to determine if the prostate cancer has spread, and, if so, to what extent.

The treatment of prostate cancer
Surgery, radiation therapy, and hormone therapy, and sometimes a combination of all three, are used to treat prostate cancer. Chemicals, other than hormones, are rarely used.

If the tumor has not yet spread beyond the gland it-self—and especially if the patient is elderly—treatment can sometimes be postponed because this type of cancer grows so slowly. If the patient is experiencing uncomfortable symptoms, however, the prostate, or at least the part that contains the tumor, can be removed.

If the tumor is localized, it can sometimes be reduced by radiation therapy.

Hormone treatment is often used when the cancer has metastasized to other parts of the body. Sometimes the testes, which produce male hormones and promote pros-tate tumor growth, are removed. Other times female hor-mones are injected to counterbalance the male hormones.

Hormone treatment for prostate cancer can produce un-pleasant side effects. Some of these drugs cause impo-tence—the loss of the ability to have sexual intercourse.

Hormone therapy can also cause the patient's breasts to become enlarged, although radiating the breasts prior to hormone therapy will generally prevent this uncomfortable side effect.

Stomach Cancer

What is the stomach?
The stomach is a muscular, pear-shaped bag that conveys food from the esophagus to the intestines. The stomach operates like a washing machine. The food is the laundry, and when it enters the stomach, gastric juices pour in like water. When the stomach churns the food, the gastric juices mix with it to form chyme, which is then digested.

What is stomach cancer?
Cancer of the stomach is a carcinoma that develops in the epithelial cells of the innermost layer of the stomach wall's three layers. The tumor spreads from this inner layer toward the outer layers. When stomach cancer metastasizes, it tends to spread through the bloodstream to the liver or lungs,

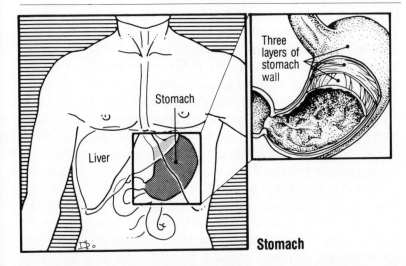

Stomach

and through the lymphatic system to the lymph nodes nearby. Sometimes stomach cancer also spreads to other nearby organs, such as the pancreas or the spleen.

At one time stomach cancer was a major cause of death in North America. Over the past couple of decades, however, the incidence of stomach cancer has declined, and it is continuing to decline.

Who gets stomach cancer and what is the outlook?

Approximately 27,600 North Americans develop cancer of the stomach each year. Almost two-thirds of these people are men, mostly over the age of fifty-five.

Cancer of the stomach is more common among people in low-income groups. Researchers speculate that this may be due to the fact that people in low-income groups tend to eat fewer fresh fruits and vegetables and more preserved foods than people in higher income brackets.

When it is detected at an early stage—before it has invaded more than two of the three layers of the stomach wall—stomach cancer can be successfully treated. Unfortunately, early detection is rare, and approximately 16,600 North Americans die of this disease every year.

About five years after treatment is stopped, surviving stomach cancer patients are considered cured.

What causes stomach cancer and who is at high risk?
While the incidence of stomach cancer has been declining in North America, it has remained high in other countries. Scientists have not been able to discover the exact reason for this, because many things about the causes of cancer are still a mystery. Most researchers, however, believe that a high use, over many years, of preservatives such as nitrates and nitrites, along with a low consumption of fresh foods, particularly fruit and vegetables containing vitamin C, increase a person's risk of developing stomach cancer.

Entire populations of countries where people's diets are high in preservatives and low in fresh fruit and vegetables have a higher-than-average risk of developing stomach cancer. Ten times as many Japanese as North Americans, for example, develop stomach cancer. The lack of refrigeration in Japan, until recently, resulted in the high use of preservatives and low use of fresh fruit and vegetables. This is the reason most scientists give for the high rate of stomach cancer in that country.

People who have had stomach surgery for ulcers or have suffered from a particular kind of anemia (called pernicious anemia), or achlorhydria (a lack of hydrochloric acid in the stomach), tend to have a higher-than-normal risk of developing stomach cancer.

The signs and symptoms of stomach cancer
One of the problems in detecting stomach cancer at an early stage is that the symptoms are usually very vague. Even by the time stomach cancer has reached an advanced stage, most people complain only of mild stomach pain, a slight feeling of nausea, or persistent heartburn. When there are more definite signs and symptoms, they are usually fatigue, vomiting, blood in the stools, or rapid weight loss.

Surveillance for stomach cancer
Because of its high rate of stomach cancer, Japan has developed better methods for early diagnosis of this disease. The Japanese now conduct mass-screening programs for stomach cancer just as we in North America conduct mass-screening programs for cancer of the cervix and the breast.

The Japanese test tens of thousands of people every year by examining their stomachs with barium X-rays. Some Japanese studies have shown that stomach cancer can be cured 95 percent of the time when it is detected at an early stage.

Because the rate of stomach cancer in North America is low, it is not practical to conduct mass-screening programs. What we could do, but don't, is to screen people who have a higher-than-average risk of developing this disease.

The diagnosis of stomach cancer

When stomach cancer is suspected, an X-ray is taken to determine if there is a tumor and its location.

If it looks as if there is a tumor, the patient is sedated, and a gastroscope is inserted through the mouth into the stomach. The doctor examines the stomach for a tumor; if there is one, a biopsy is taken.

Sometimes a tiny piece of tissue is nipped off the tumor and examined; other times cells are simply scraped off the surface of the tumor with a tiny brush. The biopsy is then sent to a lab for examination.

The treatment of stomach cancer

The treatment for stomach cancer is surgery. The tumor is removed, and part, or all, of the stomach is generally removed as well. Sometimes the spleen is removed, if it is suspected that the original tumor has spread to this nearby organ.

When it is obvious that the disease has metastasized, chemotherapy is sometimes added to the treatment in the hope of stopping, or at least slowing down, the spreading process.

Stomach cancer patients can live an almost normal life without a stomach. When the stomach has been removed, eating a number of small meals per day, rather than three large ones, will usually control digestive problems. Many cancer patients who have lost their stomachs also find that a low-carbohydrate, high-protein diet is helpful. Most people also take injections of vitamin B12.

Cancer of the Testes (Testicles)

What are the testes?

The two testes, or testicles, are the male sex organs that produce sperm, which are the cells that fertilize the female egg. They are oval-shaped organs that are suspended in a pouch, called the scrotum.

What is cancer of the testes?

Cancer of the testes, which is sometimes called testicular cancer, is a carcinoma that develops in the epithelial cells of the testicles' lining.

Testicular cancer is very scary to many men, who believe that they will automatically lose the ability to father children, or to have sexual intercourse at all. This is not usually true. Almost all cases of testicular cancer involve only one of the two organs, and a man who has only one testicle can have sex, or father children, as easily as a man with two.

Who gets cancer of the testes and what is the outlook?

Fewer than 5,400 North American men develop cancer of the testicles each year. Most of them are between the ages

Testes

of twenty-five and forty, and almost 90 percent can be cured. Approximately 550 North American men die of cancer of the testes each year.

Five years after treatment, surviving testicular cancer patients are considered cured.

What causes testicular cancer and who is at high risk?
Although the exact causes of testicular cancer are unknown, researchers have been able to show that men whose brothers or fathers have had testicular cancer are more likely to develop the disease than men in whose families there has been no history of testicular cancer.

The testes are formed inside the body near the kidneys, and normally they descend into the scrotum shortly after birth. Males whose testicles never descend, or descend after the age of six, also have a higher-than-normal risk of developing testicular cancer.

The signs and symptoms of testicular cancer
Testicular cancer is usually discovered when a swelling, or a hard lump, is noticed in a testicle. Sometimes the patient is also aware of a dull ache in the abdominal area and, if the tumor is growing quickly, there may be sharp pain. Some patients' breasts become enlarged; others develop tender nipples. The symptoms are due to a change in hormone production caused by the tumor.

The diagnosis of testicular cancer
When a testicular tumor is suspected, the doctor will first examine the testicle. If a tumor can be felt, further tests are usually performed to determine if the disease has metastasized. A blood test for this purpose has recently been developed. A biopsy is rarely taken for this type of carcinoma.

The treatment of testicular cancer
Surgery, radiation therapy, and chemotherapy are all used in the treatment of testicular cancer.

Testicular tumors are first removed surgically. Cells from them are examined to determine if they are cancerous.

Sometimes nearby lymph nodes are also surgically removed and tested.

Radiation therapy and chemotherapy are also sometimes used to treat localized testicular cancers as well as those that have spread.

Oral Cancer

What is oral cancer?
Oral cancers are a group of cancers which develop in the epithelial cells of the tissues that line the mouth: lips, gums, floor of the mouth, tongue, salivary glands, tonsils, and the back of the throat, called the pharynx. Because of their location, oral cancers are usually detected at an early stage, with the patients themselves being the best detectives. When oral cancers spread, they tend to move into the lymph nodes of the neck and sometimes into the bones nearby.

Who gets oral cancer and what is the outlook?
Approximately 31,700 North Americans develop one of the different types of oral cancer each year. Oral cancers rarely develop in young people; the vast majority of oral cancer patients are over the age of sixty.

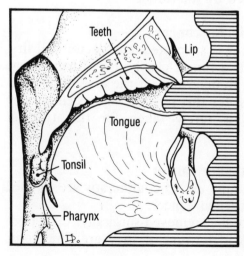

Mouth

When they are detected early, most oral cancers can be treated successfully. The approximately 10,000 North Americans who die from this disease each year are mostly those whose cancers were not detected at an early stage.

Five years after treatment is stopped, surviving oral cancer patients are considered cured.

What causes oral cancer and who is at high risk?
While the exact cause of oral cancer is unknown, scientists do know that the disease is not contagious in any way. No one has caught oral cancer from touching or kissing someone who does have it.

Studies are beginning to suggest that certain chemicals, nutrients, and hormones encourage oral cancers to develop. From studies such as these, scientists have been able to show that some people have a higher-than-normal risk of developing this disease.

People who develop cancer of the mouth, for example, are four times more likely to be smokers than non-smokers. People who smoke pipes or cigars develop lip cancer more frequently than non-smokers.

The ultraviolet rays of the sun can also cause cancer to develop on the lips. People who work or play in the sun for long periods of time can protect themselves from lip cancer by using a sunscreen containing PABA, or a sunblock containing either zinc oxide or titanium dioxide.

Heavy alcohol drinkers develop oral cancer more frequently than people who don't drink at all, or drink moderately. If a person smokes *and* drinks heavily, the chances of developing oral cancer are even higher.

Few people chew tobacco these days, but studies done in the southern U.S., where this habit is still popular, have linked it to oral cancer.

Betel-nut chewing, a habit popular among Asians, has also been linked to oral cancer.

The signs and symptoms of oral cancer
Oral cancer is not generally painful at an early stage. It usually shows up as sores that either bleed easily or don't heal properly. Sometimes a precancerous condition called

leukoplakia develops prior to an oral cancer. The signs of leukoplakia are white, or red and white, areas inside the mouth.

The diagnosis of oral cancer
Although most suspicious spots in or around the mouth turn out to be benign, any sore that persists for several weeks should be examined by a dentist or a doctor.

If a sore does look suspicious, a biopsy will be performed and cells from it will be sent to a lab for microscopic examination.

The treatment of oral cancer
Surgery or radiation therapy, and sometimes a combination of the two, are used in the treatment of oral cancer.

When radiation therapy is chosen, patients generally experience uncomfortable side effects for a number of months. They sometimes lose their sense of taste and experience a condition called dry mouth, due to the fact that radiation temporarily destroys the cells produced by the saliva glands. The teeth usually become loosened, and for this reason a dentist is generally part of the treatment team. Rest and good nutrition are particularly important for patients undergoing treatment for oral cancer.

Sometimes, if the doctor believes that an oral cancer has metastasized, the lymph nodes near the cancer site are radiated as well. There are also times when cosmetic surgery is necessary, but this is not usual. Most oral cancers are detected early enough so that there is very little scarring of the face as a result of treatment.

Cancer of the Colon and the Rectum (Colorectal Cancer)

What are the colon and the rectum?
The colon, which is also called the large intestine or large bowel, is a long, hollow organ whose job is to remove the liquid from undigested food. By the time the waste that remains gets to the final portion of the colon, called the

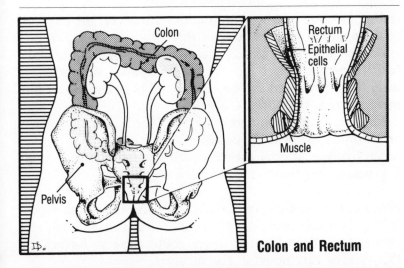

Colon

Rectum
Epithelial
cells

Muscle

Pelvis

Colon and Rectum

rectum, it is in the form that we recognize as a normal stool, or bowel movement. At the very end of the rectum is the anus, a muscular valve that can be controlled.

The wall, or lining, of the colon is made up of epithelial cells, which actually absorb this liquid. The epithelial cells also produce mucus, which lubricates the passageway. If the passageway is irritated for some reason, the epithelial cells will produce more mucus to reduce the irritation.

What is colorectal cancer?
Cancers of the colon and rectum are usually talked about as one type of cancer called colorectal cancer. They develop in the epithelial cells that line the interior of the large intestine and the rectum.

Who gets colorectal cancer and what is the outlook?
Colorectal cancer is diagnosed in about 148,000 North Americans each year, most of them over the age of fifty. Unlike many cancers that are associated with sex organs or lifestyles that are more common to either men or women, colorectal cancers develop fairly evenly among males and females.

When it is detected at an early stage, the outlook for cancer of the colon is good; 70 percent of patients can be cured. Once cancer of the colon has spread beyond the intestine into the nearby lymph nodes, however, the chances of survival fall to about one in three.

Cancer of the rectum has a less optimistic prognosis. Only half the people whose cancer of the rectum is still localized when it is diagnosed can be cured, and once the cancer has metastasized, the outlook is grim.

Each year, approximately 65,500 North American men and women die of this disease.

Surviving colorectal cancer patients are considered cured five years after treatment has been stopped.

What causes colorectal cancer and who is at high risk?
While the exact cause of colorectal cancer is unknown, scientists have been learning more about the risk factors for this type of carcinoma in recent years.

People whose diets are high in fat, and low in citrus fruit and certain vegetables like cabbage and cauliflower, tend to have a higher-than-normal risk of developing colorectal cancer. Recent studies have shown that a diet high in animal fat destroys the epithelial cells of the colon, which must then be regenerated. If calcium is added to this high-fat diet, however, these epithelial cells are not destroyed. This may possibly mean that a diet high in animal fat has a different effect than a diet high in milk fat, although no studies have as yet been conducted on humans.

Scientists believe that small, non-cancerous growths called benign polyps, which develop in the epithelial tissues of the intestines, can eventually become cancerous if they are not removed.

People who have had colorectal cancer once have a higher-than-normal risk of developing it a second time, and people whose close relatives have had this disease also seem to develop it more frequently than people with no family history of colorectal cancer. Epidemiologists are not certain whether this has to do with hereditary factors or environmental factors, such as diet, but more and more research is pointing to dietary factors.

The signs and symptoms of colorectal cancer
Most of the symptoms for colorectal cancer are the same

as the symptoms for other intestinal problems. A change in bowel habits is the most common symptom, but any bleeding, or obvious amounts of mucus in the stools, should be checked right away.

The diagnosis of colorectal cancer

When cancer of the colon or rectum is suspected, a stool sample is taken and examined for the presence of blood. Sometimes there is such a small amount of blood that it can't be detected without a chemical test. In this case it is called "occult" (the Latin word for "hidden") blood.

A barium X-ray is usually taken to determine the location of a suspected tumor. If a tumor is located, a colonoscope will be used to take a biopsy, and cells from it will be sent to a lab for examination.

Most intestinal problems do not turn out to be cancer. On the one hand, this is heartening. But many doctors worry that people who are embarrassed at the thought of an examination of the colon may use the information as an excuse to avoid checking into what might be an early cancer.

The treatment of colorectal cancer

Surgery, radiation therapy, and chemotherapy, and sometimes a combination of the three, are used to treat colorectal cancer.

Surgery is most often chosen. Resecting the colon may seem frightening, but the colon is not essential to life. If a section of the colon is removed, the two ends can be rejoined, and what remains will usually take over the organ's entire function.

If the rectum and the anus are cancerous, however, they must both be removed and a permanent colostomy performed. This means that the stools will be discharged into a plastic bag. While a procedure such as this is unpleasant to think about, many of us have met people who have colostomies and just haven't realized it. Thousands of men and women with colostomies live perfectly normal lives.

The United Ostomy Association provides advice and emotional support to people, or the families of people, who have had colostomies. A local unit of the American or the

Canadian Cancer Society can put you in touch with such a group.

Although it is not used for cancer of the colon, radiation therapy is sometimes used for cancer of the rectum. Radiation therapy can also sometimes be used before surgery to shrink a tumor, or after surgery to mop up cancerous cells that may not have been accessible to the surgeon because of the shape of the tumor.

Chemotherapy is also sometimes used in the treatment of colorectal cancer, although few of the drugs that are currently available work well for either of these two types of carcinomas.

Cancer of the Uterus

What is the uterus?
The uterus, or womb, is a pear-shaped muscular organ in which the fetus develops during pregnancy. There are two parts to the uterus: the body and the cervix. The endometrium lines the organ's hollow body, which tapers down into a narrower structure called the cervix. The cervix leads into the vagina.

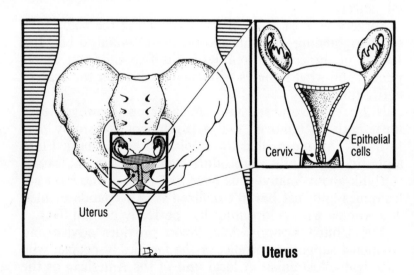

Uterus

When a woman is not pregnant, the endometrium thickens monthly and is shed during menstruation.

There are two very different types of cancer of the uterus, which is sometimes called uterine cancer: cancer of the cervix, and cancer of the endometrium.

Cancer of the Cervix

What is cancer of the cervix?
Cancer of the cervix develops in the epithelial cells that line the cervix and is sometimes called cervical cancer.

Most of the time the cells of the cervix go through mild to severe changes, often over a period of years, before the cells actually mutate enough to be called cancer. These precancerous changes are called dysplasia.

Who gets cancer of the cervix and what is the outlook?
Cancer of the cervix, including in situ cervical cancer, is diagnosed in approximately 61,500 North American women each year, most of them between the ages of forty and forty-nine. Cancer of the cervix used to be rare among women under the age of forty, but in recent years more North American women in their thirties and even twenties have been developing this disease.

The cure rate for early cervical cancer is almost 100 percent. Most of the 7,400 North American women who die each year from this disease were diagnosed after it had already progressed to an advanced stage.

Surviving cervical cancer patients are considered cured five years after treatment has finished.

What causes cancer of the cervix and who is at high risk?
Although scientists do not know the exact cause of cervical cancer, they have been able to discover who has a higher-than-normal risk of developing it. Women who begin their sex lives early, and women who have had many partners,

are more likely to develop cervical cancer than other women.

There is some speculation as to why. The cells that line the cervical canal of a pre-adolescent female resemble columns, and are called columnar cells. The cells that line the vagina, on the other hand, are shaped differently, and are called squamous cells. These cells meet at the squamo-columnar junction, and it is at this junction that most cancers of the cervix appear. During late adolescence, the columnar cells at the squamo-columnar junction are replaced by squamous cells. Researchers have speculated that while this change is taking place, women are more susceptible to genetic mutations. They also believe that the chance of a gene becoming mutated may increase when a woman has multiple sex partners who can introduce a virus or possibly other carcinogens to the area.

The signs and symptoms of cervical cancer
The first signs of cervical cancer are bleeding, often after sexual intercourse, or vaginal discharge. When cervical cancer is at a very early stage, however, there are usually no symptoms at all.

The diagnosis of cervical cancer
Cancer of the cervix can be diagnosed at an early stage by a simple, painless procedure called the Pap test, which is described in detail on page 46.

The Pap test can detect dysplasia as well as early cancer. If there is any unusual bleeding or discharge from the cervix, or if the results of a Pap test are positive, the doctor will perform a type of endoscopy. Using a colposcope, the physician can examine the cervix for suspicious-looking tissue. If there is any, a biopsy will be taken, and cells from it will be sent to a lab for microscopic examination.

The treatment of cervical cancer
If the biopsy indicates dysplasia, the doctor might simply decide to keep a close watch on the patient to see if these changes reverse themselves, which they sometimes do.

If the cells are severely dysplasic, or clearly cancerous,

a conization is frequently performed. A cone-shaped sample of tissue about a centimeter thick is resected surgically from the entire length of the cervix. Usually it is only necessary to remain in hospital for a day or two after a conization is performed, and there is only mild discomfort for a few days after that. A conization rarely affects a woman's sex life or her ability to bear children.

Sometimes, when the doctor suspects that there are abnormal cells farther along the cervix than can be seen with a colposcope, a conization will be performed as a preventive measure. The cells that are removed when a conization is performed also provide a better sample for the biopsy than do cells from a Pap test or a colposcope biopsy.

Sometimes abnormal areas of the cervix are treated by cryosurgery, which destroys tissue by freezing it. Other times cancer cells are destroyed by heat. A new treatment is laser beam surgery. All three of these techniques can be performed in a doctor's office, with no general anesthetic. They are only mildly uncomfortable and, like the conization, only rarely affect a woman's sex life or her ability to bear children.

On occasion, if a woman is not interested in having children and the doctor suspects that the disease may have spread, a hysterectomy will be performed. This is the surgical resection of the entire cervix, the uterus, and sometimes the fallopian tubes as well.

When cancer of the cervix is more advanced, the treatment is more complicated.

Usually radiation therapy is chosen and, occasionally, the doctor will combine radiation therapy with surgery.

When radiation therapy is chosen, both internal and external radiation are usually used. To radiate internally, radioactive pellets are inserted into the uterus for several days. Hospitalization is necessary during this time. External radiation can usually be performed without a hospital stay.

If radiotherapy is not successful, radical surgery is occasionally possible. On rare occasions, chemotherapy, which is considered experimental for cervical cancer, is used.

Endometrial Cancer

What is endometrial cancer?
Endometrial cancer develops in the endometrium, or lining, of the body of the uterus.

The cells of the endometrium go through pre-cancerous changes called hyperplasia before they become abnormal enough to be called cancerous.

Who gets endometrial cancer and what is the outlook?
Endometrial cancer is diagnosed in approximately 33,300 North American women each year, most of them between the ages of fifty and sixty-five. Approximately 3,400 North American women die from this type of cancer each year.

Early endometrial cancer can be successfully treated approximately 75 percent of the time. This rate could be as high as 90 percent if women recognized the symptoms of endometrial cancer and consulted a doctor immediately.

Five years after treatment is finished, surviving endometrial cancer patients are considered cured.

What causes endometrial cancer and who is at high risk?
Although the exact cause of endometrial cancer is unknown, studies have shown that certain women between the ages of fifty and sixty-five have a higher-than-normal risk of developing this type of carcinoma. These are women who are overweight, diabetic, show signs of hypertension, have uterine bleeding after they have stopped menstruating, or continue to have periods after the age of fifty. Women who have never borne children and women who take hormones, other than birth control pills, also have a higher-than-normal risk of developing this disease.

Only half the women who do develop endometrial cancer are in these high-risk groups, however, and all women should be aware of the symptoms of endometrial cancer.

The signs and symptoms of endometrial cancer
The most common sign of endometrial cancer is unusual bleeding. For post-menopausal women, this means any sort of bleeding; for women who are still menstruating, this means excessive bleeding during periods, or bleeding between periods.

The diagnosis of endometrial cancer
There are two types of tests for endometrial cancer. They are the aspiration curettage and the dilation and curettage of the uterus, usually referred to as a "D and C."

The aspiration curettage is a simple procedure, which can be performed in a doctor's office without a general anesthetic. A thin tube is inserted through the cervix into the body of the uterus. Suction is used to take a biopsy, which is sent to a lab for examination.

A general anesthetic is necessary to do a D and C. The cervix is stretched, or dilated, and a tiny instrument is inserted into the uterine body. Cells from the lining of the body are then scraped off, or curettaged, and this biopsy is sent to a lab for examination.

The treatment of endometrial cancer
If very mild pre-cancerous changes are detected in the cells of the endometrium, the woman is usually watched carefully rather than treated; often these changes will reverse themselves. More serious cell changes often respond to hormone therapy. Drugs that bring on a menstrual period are taken, and the endometrium is shed along with the abnormal cells.

When cancerous cells are discovered, however, a hysterectomy must usually be performed. The entire uterus, the fallopian tubes, and sometimes the lymph nodes nearby are surgically removed. In some cases radiation therapy is added to the treatment. Sometimes internal radiation is chosen; other times external radiation is given.

If the doctor suspects that the cancer has metastasized to other parts of the body, chemotherapy will generally be added to the treatment.

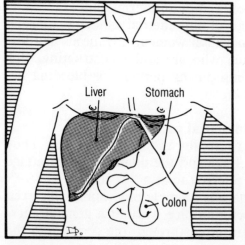

Liver

Cancer of the Liver

What is the liver?
The liver is a complex organ that fills the upper right side of the abdomen and is protected by the rib cage.

The functions of the liver are too numerous to list completely, but they include: converting worn-out red blood cells into bile, producing proteins essential to blood clotting, and storing sugar and some vitamins.

What is cancer of the liver?
Most cancers of the liver are secondary tumors that have spread to the liver from other organs. Sometimes, however, primary liver cancer does develop in the epithelial cells of this organ.

Who gets liver cancer and what is the outlook?
Liver cancer is diagnosed in approximately 13,800 North Americans each year. Because it is seldom detected at an early stage, this type of carcinoma can rarely be treated successfully, and almost everyone who has been diagnosed with liver cancer will die of the disease.

What causes liver cancer and who is at high risk?
The exact cause of liver cancer is unknown, but studies have shown that exposure to certain chemicals, such as vinyl chloride, can increase a person's risk of developing this disease.

Athletes, such as weight lifters, who have taken large amounts of testosterone to increase their strength also have a higher-than-normal risk of developing liver cancer.

The signs and symptoms of liver cancer
There are no symptoms of liver cancer until the disease has progressed to an advanced stage. Even then they are the same vague symptoms that others with cancers in organs deep in the abdomen complain of: mild discomfort, weakness, or loss of appetite.

The diagnosis of liver cancer
When liver cancer is suspected, X-rays are first taken to determine if there is a tumor. But, to confirm the diagnosis, a biopsy must be performed. A local anesthetic is given first, and then a needle is inserted through the skin into the liver to obtain some tumor cells. These cells will be sent to a lab for microscopic examination.

If a diagnosis of liver cancer is confirmed, tests will be performed to determine if the cancer has spread.

The treatment of liver cancer
Radiation therapy or chemotherapy can sometimes extend the life of a patient who has cancer of the liver. Most care for liver cancer is palliative, however, since it cannot be cured.

Cancer of the Bladder

What is the bladder?
The bladder is a muscular "balloon" that stores urine. The kidneys process the urine, and from there it goes down a tube called the ureter to the bladder. From the bladder the

Bladder

urine goes down another tube, called the urethra, and then leaves the body.

What is cancer of the bladder?
Bladder cancer develops in the epithelial cells of the bladder's inner lining. Most bladder cancer tumors are "papillary" tumors; they look like tiny mushrooms whose stems are attached to the organ's lining. Some papillary tumors are benign rather than cancerous.

A less common type of bladder cancer, called epidermoid carcinoma, grows directly on the lining of the bladder and tends to invade the organ's muscular wall.

Who gets cancer of the bladder and what is the outlook?
Bladder cancer is diagnosed in approximately 43,200 North Americans each year. The majority are men over the age of fifty; only one in three bladder cancer patients is a woman.

When it is diagnosed at an early stage, cancer of the bladder can be successfully treated. Approximately 11,800

North Americans die each year of bladder cancer that was invasive by the time it was detected.

Five years after treatment is discontinued, surviving bladder cancer patients are considered cured.

What causes bladder cancer and who is at high risk?
Although the exact cause of bladder cancer is unknown, certain people have a higher-than-normal risk of developing this type of cancer. Studies have shown that exposure to certain industrial chemicals such as beta-napthylamine can increase a person's risk of bladder cancer. Other studies have linked tobacco, alcohol, and tea and coffee in large amounts over many years, to cancer of the bladder.

The signs and symptoms of bladder cancer
There is usually no pain associated with cancer of the bladder; the first sign is blood in the urine.

Blood in the urine is certainly not a sure sign of bladder cancer. If cancer of the bladder is suspected, a number of diagnostic tests must be done.

The diagnosis of bladder cancer
When a bladder tumor is suspected, the urine is analyzed to see if it contains any cancerous cells. The second test is a type of endoscopy. A cystoscope inserted into the bladder is used to locate and snip off a piece of the tumor. These cells are sent to a lab for microscopic examination. Sometimes, the entire tumor can be removed during the endoscopy procedure.

The treatment of bladder cancer
If the tumor cells are cancerous, radiation therapy or surgery will generally be used. Chemotherapy is sometimes used when the disease has metastasized to other parts of the body.

A single papillary tumor can often be removed with a cystoscope. Instead of biopsying a section of the tumor incisionally, the doctor will remove it entirely—this is called an excisional biopsy.

When there are several tumors, more extensive surgery is necessary. The tumors, as well as a margin of normal tissue, will be removed.

Radiation therapy is sometimes used as an alternative to surgery. With modern high-voltage radiation equipment, X-rays can be directed at tumors in the bladder without permanent damage to other tissue. In Vancouver, at the B.C. Cancer Research Centre, experiments are also being conducted on bladder cancer patients using pion beams. The initial results look promising.

In a few cases, a cystectomy, a surgical procedure to remove the entire bladder, must be performed. In this case a bag must be used to collect urine. The idea of living without a bladder sounds much worse than it really is. The United Ostomy Association, which was formed to assist people without colons, also provides information and emotional support to people who have had their bladders surgically removed. A local unit of the American or Canadian Cancer Society can put you in touch with a nearby branch.

Cancer of the Ovary

What are the ovaries?
The ovaries are the female reproductive organs in which the ova, or eggs, are formed. During the menstrual cycle, an egg is discharged from one of the ovaries and travels to the uterus by way of a fallopian tube. The ovaries also release the female hormone estrogen. When a woman gets to the age of about forty-eight, the ovaries begin to produce less estrogen. At first the menstrual periods become irregular, and then they stop completely. This is called menopause, and women who have stopped menstruating are sometimes referred to as post-menopausal women.

What is cancer of the ovaries?
Cancer of the ovaries, which is sometimes called ovarian cancer, develops in the epithelial cells that line the ovaries. Usually only one of the two organs is affected.

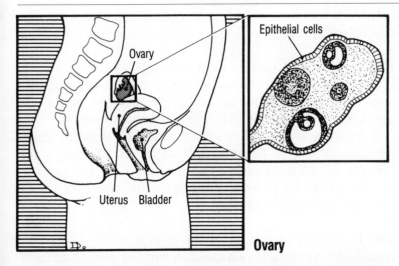

Ovary

Who gets cancer of the ovary and what is the outlook?

Ovarian cancer is diagnosed in approximately 20,000 North American women each year, most of whom are over the age of fifty. Most of these women cannot be successfully treated unless the disease has been diagnosed at an early stage, which is rare. Each year, approximately 12,600 North American women die of cancer of an ovary.

Five years after treatment, surviving ovarian cancer patients are considered cured.

What causes cancer of the ovary and who is at high risk?

While the exact cause of ovarian cancer is unknown, some studies have shown that women who have had a close relative with ovarian cancer have a higher-than-normal risk of developing this disease. Other studies show that women who are infertile also have a higher-than-normal risk of developing ovarian cancer. Studies to relate ovarian cancer to dietary habits are also being conducted.

The signs and symptoms of cancer of the ovary

Because the ovaries are located deep within the pelvis, there are rarely any symptoms—no pain, no bleeding, and no obvious swelling—until the disease has progressed to an advanced stage. When it is discovered at an early stage, it is usually by chance during an examination for some un-related problem.

The diagnosis of cancer of the ovary
If cancer of the ovary is suspected, a number of diagnostic tests are performed. X-rays and ultrasound are used to determine the size and location of a suspected tumor.

If a tumor is located, a minor surgical procedure called laparoscopy will be performed. This involves cutting a tiny "peephole" in the abdomen so that a biopsy of the ovary can be taken. Cells from the biopsy are sent to a lab for microscopic examination.

The treatment of cancer of the ovary
If an ovarian tumor is cancerous, a surgical procedure called an oophorectomy will be performed. Both ovaries, the fallopian tubes, and the uterus are generally removed, whether or not it is suspected that the tumor has metastasized.

If it is obvious that the cancer has spread, radiation therapy, or chemotherapy, and sometimes both, can be used.

Cancer of the Pancreas

What is the pancreas?
The pancreas is a gland that is located behind the stomach. It produces proteins, which help digest food, and insulin, which regulates the amount of sugar in the blood.

What is cancer of the pancreas?
Most cancers of the pancreas develop in the cells that make up the organ's duct system. Occasionally, however, cancer of the pancreas begins in the cells that produce insulin, the Islets of Langerhans.

Who gets cancer of the pancreas and what is the outlook?
Every year, approximately 26,200 North Americans de-

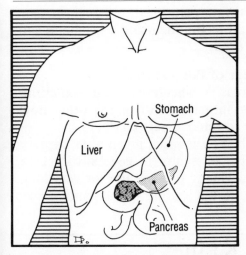

Pancreas

velop cancer of the pancreas. Few patients with this type of carcinoma survive.

What causes cancer of the pancreas and who is at high risk?
Some studies have linked cancer of the pancreas with cigarette smoking, although scientists do not understand why.

The signs and symptoms of cancer of the pancreas
Cancer of the pancreas is rarely discovered at an early stage. There are no symptoms—no pain or swelling—until it has advanced, and by that time a patient will usually only notice a vague pain in the abdomen or back. Sometimes there is weight loss, nausea, or a feeling of general weakness.

The diagnosis of cancer of the pancreas
When cancer of the pancreas is suspected, a barium X-ray is taken; when barium is swallowed prior to an X-ray, a much clearer picture of the organ can be obtained.

Recently, doctors in some hospitals have been using CT scans or ultrasound to locate tumors in the pancreas and to determine their size.

When it has been established that there is a tumor, a biopsy will be taken to determine if its cells are cancerous. To do a biopsy of the pancreas, a surgical procedure called a laparotomy is almost always performed, although in some hospitals a minor surgical technique using a needle to suction cells is sometimes used.

The treatment of cancer of the pancreas

If a tumor in the pancreas is cancerous, it can sometimes be removed entirely by surgery. Most of the time, however, it is only possible to remove part of it.

Radiation or chemotherapy is often given after surgery, and while these two types of treatment generally decrease discomfort, they do not usually prolong life for very long. If there is pain, certain nerves leading to the pancreas can sometimes be blocked.

Cancer of the Kidney

What are the kidneys?

The kidneys are a pair of organs that are located behind the liver and stomach near the spine, one on either side. The kidneys help to remove wastes from the body by manufacturing urine. They do this by filtering urea, salt, and other substances from the blood as it flows through them. Three tubes enter each kidney at the point where the organ indents: the renal vein, the renal artery, and the

Kidney

ureter, which is the long tube down which urine flows to the bladder. The shell enclosing the kidney is called the capsule. Inside the kidney, blood is filtered by thousands of filament-like tubes called renal tubules. The renal pelvis collects the urine that is produced, and funnels it into the ureter.

The kidneys also manufacture and secrete a variety of hormones.

There are two very different types of kidney cancer. One occurs in adults; the other almost always occurs in children and is called Wilm's tumor. Wilm's tumor is one of the only types of carcinomas that affect children; most children who develop cancer are afflicted with a form of leukemia, lymphoma, or sarcoma.

Adult Cancer of the Kidney

What is cancer of the kidney in adults?
Most of the time, cancer of the kidney in adults develops in the cells that form the lining of a renal tubule. In rare cases a tumor will begin to grow on the renal capsule itself.

Who gets adult kidney cancer and what is the outlook?
Kidney cancer is diagnosed in approximately 20,700 North American adults each year, most of whom are over the age of forty. Almost twice as many males develop kidney cancer as females. Less than a third of the adults who develop this disease can be successfully treated; approximately 9,500 adult North Americans die of kidney cancer each year.

Five years after treatment is finished, surviving adult kidney cancer patients are considered cured.

What causes adult kidney cancer and who is at high risk?
The causes of adult kidney cancer are unknown, but certain people are considered to have a higher-than-normal risk

of developing this disease. Some studies show that people who smoke have a higher-than-normal risk of developing kidney cancer, and studies that may link certain dietary habits to kidney cancer are now being conducted.

The signs and symptoms of adult kidney cancer
Kidney cancer in adults is sometimes suspected because of blood in the urine, although this can also be the sign of many urinary disorders other than cancer.

Other times patients will feel a lump in the abdomen and vague pain. Some people with kidney cancer complain of weight loss or fatigue, but because these symptoms are common to so many other medical problems, the disease often remains undetected until it has reached an advanced stage.

The diagnosis of adult kidney cancer
When cancer of the kidney is suspected, dye to highlight the kidneys is injected into the bloodstream, and then an X-ray is taken. CT scans and ultrasound are also used sometimes to get a better idea of the size of the tumor and its exact location.

If the doctor suspects that the cancer has metastasized, bone scans or chest X-rays will be taken in an attempt to pinpoint the metastases. Most often, kidney cancer in adults will spread to the lungs and bones first.

The treatment of adult kidney cancer
When a cancerous kidney tumor is still localized, and the second kidney is working well, the cancerous kidney, a section of normal tissue, and the lymph nodes nearby will most likely be removed. This type of operation is called a nephrectomy. Because a remaining kidney will take over the function that was performed by the two organs, a person can lead a normal life with one kidney.

Sometimes radiation therapy is used before this type of surgery to shrink the tumor. Other times it is used after surgery to mop up any cancerous cells that were not able to be surgically removed.

Radiation therapy is generally used when kidney cancer has metastasized. When it has spread to the bones, radiation will often relieve the pain caused by the secondary tumor. In some cases chemotherapy is given, but anti-cancer drugs for this type of cancer are still considered experimental.

Kidney Cancer in Children— Wilm's Tumor

What is Wilm's tumor?
Wilm's tumor, which is sometimes referred to as nephroblastoma, develops in the epithelial cells that line the kidney. This type of carcinoma rarely affects both kidneys.

Who gets Wilm's tumor and what is the outlook?
Approximately 670 North American children, most of them between the ages of one and eight, are diagnosed with Wilm's tumor each year. Due to recent advances in chemotherapy, more than 75 percent of them can be treated successfully.

What causes Wilm's tumor and who is at high risk?
The exact causes of Wilm's tumor are unknown, but certain children have a higher-than-normal risk of developing this disease.

If one child in a family has had Wilm's tumor, a second child will have a higher-than-normal risk of developing the disease and will be monitored carefully. Children whose eyes lack an iris (the colored portion of the eye) also have a higher-than-average risk of developing Wilm's tumor, as do children with other developmental abnormalities.

The signs and symptoms of Wilm's tumor
The most common symptom of Wilm's tumor is a lump in the belly, or a swollen abdomen. Approximately 25 per-

cent of Wilm's tumor patients produce blood in the urine, but often the amount is so small that it can only be detected by a chemical test. The symptoms of many children are vague: low fever, fatigue, loss of appetite, weight loss, and anemia.

The diagnosis of Wilm's tumor
The diagnostic procedure for Wilm's tumor is the same as for adult cancer of the kidney, which is described on page 156.

The treatment of Wilm's tumor
Surgery, radiation therapy, chemotherapy, and sometimes a combination of all three, are used in the treatment of Wilm's tumor.

When a kidney is removed by surgery, the operation is called a nephrectomy. Usually Wilm's tumor affects only one kidney and a child can lead a normal life even if a kidney is removed. When it affects both kidneys, one tumor is usually very small. In these rare situations, one kidney and the small tumor on the second kidney can generally be removed, without removing the entire second organ.

Radiation therapy is often used after surgery to guard against recurrence. Sometimes, if a tumor is very large, it will be shrunk by radiation therapy before surgery. Radiation therapy is not used on children under the age of two.

Chemotherapy is also used in almost all cases of Wilm's tumor, and this type of treatment accounts for the fact that eight out of ten children with Wilm's tumor can be successfully treated.

The Lymphomas

Lymphomas are cancers of the lymphocytes, the white blood cells of the lymphatic system.

Hodgkin's Disease and Non-Hodgkin's Lymphoma

What is the lymphatic system?
The lymphatic system is made up of several parts. A network of vessels—similar to blood vessels—transports the colorless lymphatic fluid, called lymph, around the body; lymph bathes all of the body's cells to prevent them from drying out. At different points along the route are lymph nodes, which act as filters to sift out impurities, such as bacteria, that the lymph picks up. These nodes are made up of clusters of infection-fighting white blood cells called T and B lymphocytes.

What is cancer of the lymphatic system?
Lymphoma is the general term for cancers that develop in the tissue of the lymphatic system. It is the lymphocyte cells, which form the lymph nodes, that become cancerous.

Basically there are two types of lymphomas. One is Hodgkin's disease. The other is non-Hodgkin's lym-

The Lymphatic System

phoma. Both are cancers of the lymphatic system, but they differ in several ways.

In Hodgkin's disease, particular cells called Reed-Sternberg cells can always be found when the patient's lymph nodes are examined microscopically. With non-Hodgkin's lymphoma, there are no Reed-Sternberg cells.

As lymphomas progress, more and more cancerous lymphocyte cells are produced, leaving fewer and fewer normal cells to fight infection. For this reason lymphoma patients often develop various types of infections.

Who gets cancer of the lymphatic system and what is the outlook?

Hodgkin's disease is diagnosed in about 7,900 North Americans each year. About 28,300 people develop non-Hodgkin's lymphoma.

The majority of Hodgkin's disease patients are between the ages of twenty and forty, although this type of cancer sometimes develops in people as young as ten and as old as seventy.

The majority of people with non-Hodgkin's lymphoma are between the ages of fifty-five and seventy, although children sometimes develop this disease.

Approximately 80 percent of Hodgkin's disease patients can be successfully treated. As recently as twenty years ago, only 20 percent of these patients could be cured. Today approximately 1,700 North Americans die each year of this type of lymphoma.

The success rate for the treatment of non-Hodgkin's lymphoma is not as high. Approximately 14,600 North Americans die each year from non-Hodgkin's lymphoma.

When they have been off treatment for eight years, surviving lymphoma patients are considered cured.

What causes lymphoma and who is at high risk?

Although the exact cause of lymphoma is unknown, a growing number of researchers believe that people who develop this type of cancer have some sort of defect in their immune system. This defect makes them less able to fight off a certain type of virus if they are exposed to it.

Lymphomas are less common among people who have grown up in underdeveloped countries, where they have been exposed to disease during childhood. When people are exposed to a disease and survive it, they often become immune to that disease, meaning that their bodies have produced antibodies that protect them from developing the disease again. This is the reason why people develop chicken pox only once.

The signs and symptoms of lymphoma
The first sign of a lymphoma is usually a painless, swollen lymph node in the neck, armpit, or groin; a painful, inflamed node is usually not a symptom of cancer.

Occasionally there is swelling, fever, sweating, shortness of breath, back pain, unexplained weight loss, unexplained itchiness, or nausea. But since these are also the symptoms of dozens of other medical problems, lymphomas can remain undetected for some time.

The diagnosis of lymphoma
If there is something suspicious about a lymph node, it will be surgically removed and studied in a lab. If the cells are cancerous, tests to determine the extent to which the cancer has spread will be performed.

Chest X-rays are taken to see if the lymphoma has spread into the chest area. Blood tests are taken, and a lymphangiography is also performed. During a lymphangiography, a type of dye that is impervious to X-rays is injected into the lymphatic system. When the X-ray is taken, the lymphatic system is outlined and the doctor can see the extent to which the disease has spread.

If it is suspected that the disease has spread to other parts of the body, a CT scan, a bone marrow test, and biopsies of suspected organs will be taken.

The treatment of lymphoma
Because lymphomas are systemic diseases—diseases that spread throughout a system—surgery is rarely used. Radiation therapy or chemotherapy, and sometimes a combination of the two, are more often used.

Radiation therapy is usually the treatment for a lymphoma that is not widely spread.

Chemotherapy alone, or in combination with radiotherapy, is chosen when it has been determined that the disease has spread.

Multiple Myeloma

What is multiple myeloma?
Multiple myeloma, like the other lymphomas, is a cancer of the white blood cells. Lymphomas, however, are cancers of the lymphocytes, while multiple myeloma involves plasma cells, which develop from B lymphocytes and then move to the bone marrow where they are stored.

When a person develops myeloma, too many plasma cells are produced. What's worse, these plasma cells are not mature. They are unable to perform their job of producing antibodies to fight infection. They do produce antibodies—too many, in fact—but they are abnormal. They pour into the bloodstream and the lymphatic system, where they interfere with the body's normal functions.

Multiple myeloma patients also sometimes develop diseases, such as pneumonia or kidney infections, because they have lost the ability to produce the antibodies that can fight infection.

Who gets multiple myeloma and what is the outlook?
Every year, approximately 10,500 North Americans develop multiple myeloma. Most of them are over the age of fifty. Due to recent developments in chemotherapy, remissions can be achieved for many of these patients. Unfortunately, these remissions rarely last for more than a few years.

What causes multiple myeloma and who is at high risk?
The causes of multiple myeloma are unknown, although a few studies have shown that people who have been exposed to excessive amounts of radiation have a higher-than-normal risk of developing this disease.

The signs and symptoms of multiple myeloma

Multiple myeloma is usually discovered when a person has pain in the bones. This is caused by the abnormal number of plasma cells in the bone marrow. Sometimes multiple myeloma patients complain of fatigue, because the abnormal plasma cells are interfering with the production of red blood cells that carry oxygen to the body. Some people suffer from nosebleeds, bleeding gums, or bruising, because fewer platelets, which control bleeding, are produced.

The diagnosis of multiple myeloma

When multiple myeloma is suspected, X-rays are taken to locate the tumor.

Since cancerous plasma cells produce abnormal proteins, which are eventually excreted in the urine, multiple myeloma is one of the few cancers that can sometimes be diagnosed through a urine sample.

The conclusive test for multiple myeloma, however, is a bone marrow aspiration and usually a bone biopsy is taken as well.

For the bone marrow aspiration, an area on either the breastbone or the pelvis is anesthetized, and a thin needle is inserted into the marrow of the bone. A small bit of tissue is then suctioned out, and cells from it are sent to a lab for microscopic examination. The aspiration procedure is usually painful, but only for a brief moment.

The treatment of multiple myeloma

Chemotherapy is most often used to treat multiple myeloma. Sometimes radiation therapy is also used, because it can shrink collections of cancerous cells, enabling the body to repair the bone damage that myeloma can cause. Radiation therapy can also relieve pain caused by multiple myeloma.

When a multiple myeloma patient is in remission, bone marrow aspirations, blood tests, and urine samples are taken frequently to ensure that the patient does not go out of remission undetected.

The Leukemias

What is leukemia?

The word "leukemia" literally means "white blood." Leukemias are cancers of various types of leukocytes, or white blood cells, that are produced in the bone marrow.

If you've read the sections on lymphomas and multiple myeloma, you may be a bit confused.

When a person develops lymphoma, specific white blood cells of the lymphatic system, called T and B lymphocytes, become cancerous.

When a person develops multiple myeloma, white blood cells called plasma cells, which are stored in bone marrow, become cancerous. Plasma cells actually develop from B lymphocytes.

The bone marrow itself also produces blood cells. Red blood cells, for example, normally deliver oxygen to body tissues; white blood cells called granulocytes (or polys) fight infection in the bloodstream; and platelets control and prevent bleeding.

When a person develops leukemia, too many abnormal white blood cells are produced. Eventually, these immature white blood cells monopolize the bone marrow, which then produces too few red blood cells, and insufficient platelets.

Who gets leukemia and what is the outlook?

Leukemia is usually thought of as a childhood disease because the treatment of childhood leukemia, which is one of the great success stories of cancer therapy, has received a great deal of publicity. More adults than children, however, are affected by leukemia.

Each year, one of the various types of leukemia is diagnosed in approximately 26,500 North American adults. Acute myelogenous leukemia, usually called AML, is the most common type of adult leukemia. Leukemia is more difficult to treat successfully in adults than in children; almost 18,500 adults die of this type of cancer every year.

Approximately 950 North American children are diagnosed with leukemia each year, the majority of whom develop acute lymphoblastic leukemia, or ALL. More than half these children can be treated successfully.

The overall cure rate for all people with all types of leukemia, however, is only about 20 percent. Although leukemia patients must survive for five years after treatment to be considered cured, it is unusual for a patient to go out of remission two years after treatment is finished.

What causes leukemia and who is at high risk?

The exact causes of leukemia are unknown, but researchers have been able to show that certain people have a higher-than-normal risk of developing this kind of cancer.

Excessive exposure to radiation or certain drugs increases a person's risk of developing leukemia. Some patients who are treated for other kinds of cancer, such as Hodgkin's disease, cancer of the ovary, or multiple myeloma, develop leukemia a number of years later.

The signs and symptoms of leukemia

Sometimes leukemia is detected when the bone marrow's overproduction of abnormal white blood cells interferes with the production of red blood cells. When there are too few red blood cells, too little oxygen will be delivered to the body's cells, and the patient will complain of fatigue.

Other times leukemia is discovered because too few platelets are being produced. In this case the signs will be bruising, frequent nosebleeds, or bleeding of the gums.

In still other cases leukemia is suspected because the leukemic white blood cells are not able to fight infection, and something as minor as a sore throat will not improve.

The diagnosis of leukemia

When there are suspicious symptoms, two diagnostic tests are usually performed.

One is a simple test, where blood is taken from a vein in the finger or arm and tested to reveal the presence of cancerous blood cells.

The other test is a bone marrow aspiration. First, a local anesthetic is injected into the hip. Then a thin needle is inserted into the marrow of the hipbone. A tiny amount of marrow is removed by suction, and cells from it are sent to the lab for examination. A bone marrow aspiration is usually painful, but only for a brief moment.

The treatment of leukemia

The objective of the treatment for leukemia is to destroy the cancerous white blood cells and increase the production of the normal types of blood cells.

Chemotherapy in two phases is used to treat leukemia. The first phase generally lasts for several months and causes more adverse side effects than the second phase. This second phase is called maintenance therapy and generally lasts for about two years. (See pages 82–83.)

Sometimes a single drug is used during the first phase of treatment, but more often a combination of cancer-killing chemicals is administered to the patient over a period of months. Doctors have achieved remissions in a high percentage of patients with leukemia. When a patient is in remission, all or at least part of the signs of the disease will disappear.

During maintenance therapy, most patients can live a fairly normal life, except perhaps for the few days a month when strong anti-cancer drugs are given.

Most adults with acute leukemia do not remain in remission for more than a few months or years. Many children, on the other hand, have been in remission for as long as fifteen years, and are considered cured.

Chemotherapy kills almost all the bone marrow cells. Because bone marrow cells reproduce very quickly, they soon increase to the normal number. If the treatment is successful, the new bone marrow cells will be normal instead of leukemic.

After the first phase of chemotherapy is finished, radiation therapy is also sometimes used to treat certain types of leukemia. The purpose of radiation therapy is to kill any leukemic cells that have spread to the brain. Many anti-cancer chemicals do not reach the brain, because of what is called the blood-brain barrier; this barrier prevents chemicals from moving into the brain from the bloodstream. Radiation to the brain, however, will often mop up the cancer cells that have been missed by chemotherapy.

An experimental type of treatment for acute leukemia is yielding some preliminary results that seem promising. It is called bone marrow transplantation, and it seems to work best on patients who are under the age of forty.

A bone marrow transplantation can be used only when there is a suitable person to donate bone marrow to the leukemia patient. That person must be someone, usually a brother or sister, whose cells have the same HLA markers (see page 21) as the leukemia patient's cells. If these markers are different, the patient's body will perceive the donated marrow as alien and reject it.

Prior to a bone marrow transplantation, all the bone marrow cells of the leukemia patient are destroyed by very strong chemicals. Then, about 500 milliliters of bone marrow is removed by suction from the hipbone of the donor while he or she is under general anesthetic. It is not a painful procedure, but usually the donor's hip area will be sore for a few days. In fact, bone marrow is extracted from the donor by the same procedure that is used to aspirate bone marrow from a leukemia patient for testing, except that more marrow is required for a transplant than for a diagnostic test.

The marrow is then administered to the leukemia patient in basically the same way as a blood transfusion. The hope is that the patient's body will accept the donor's bone marrow and begin producing normal blood cells.

Patients in remission are usually put on maintenance drug therapy, sometimes for several years, in the hope of ensuring that leukemic cells do not reappear.

The Sarcomas

Sarcomas are cancers of mesodermal cells: bone, muscle, cartilage, tendon, and ligament cells, which form supportive and connective tissues. Bone tissue is most often involved in these types of cancer.

Osteogenic Sarcoma

What is osteogenic sarcoma?
Osteogenic sarcoma is the most common form of the sarcomas, which are very rare. Osteogenic sarcoma develops in bone itself, rather than in bone marrow, which is where leukemia and multiple myeloma develop.

Most bone cancers have spread from another organ and are therefore secondary, rather than primary, cancers. There are, however, a number of different types of primary bone cancer, the most common of which is osteogenic sarcoma. This type of bone cancer can develop in long bones, flat bones, the pelvis, or the spine. Long bones, however, are the most common site for this uncommon disease. Senator Edward M. Kennedy's son, Edward M. Kennedy, Jr., was cured of this disease.

Who gets bone cancer and what is the outlook?
Fewer than 800 North Americans develop osteogenic sarcoma each year; most who do are under the age of twenty. Only a few years ago this type of cancer was fatal for eight out of ten patients. Today, however, because of advances in chemotherapy, approximately 60 percent of osteogenic sarcoma patients can be successfully treated. Because it spreads very quickly through the bloodstream, osteogenic sarcoma must be diagnosed at an early stage in order for treatment to be successful.

Five years after treatment, surviving osteogenic sarcoma patients are considered cured.

What causes osteogenic sarcoma and who is at high risk?

The causes and risk factors for this type of cancer are unknown.

The signs and symptoms of osteogenic sarcoma

The first sign of this type of cancer is usually pain in the bone where the tumor is located, followed by swelling.

The diagnosis of osteogenic sarcoma

Bone scans can determine the location of osteogenic tumors, but in order to confirm that the tumor cells are cancerous, a biopsy must be performed. A fragment of the tumor is surgically removed and sent to a lab for microscopic examination.

The treatment of osteogenic sarcoma

Surgery or radiation therapy, followed by chemotherapy, is usually used to treat osteogenic sarcoma. Usually the affected limb is amputated, although recently some research centers have been experimenting with radiation therapy so that the affected limb can be saved.

After surgery, chemotherapy is given to kill any cancer cells that may have already metastasized. Because of recent advances in anti-cancer drugs, 60 percent of patients with osteogenic sarcoma are now able to be successfully treated.

Cancer of the Brain

What is brain cancer?
Primary cancers do begin in the brain, but it is far more common for cancer to metastasize to the brain from other organs. On the other hand, cancers that develop in the tissues of the brain rarely spread to other parts of the body.

Who gets brain cancer and what is the outlook?
Approximately 15,000 North Americans develop primary brain cancer each year. Approximately 600 of these people are children. Few brain cancer patients can be successfully treated, and more than 11,000 primary brain cancer patients die each year.

What causes brain cancer and who is at high risk?
The causes and risk factors for this type of cancer are unknown.

The signs and symptoms of brain cancer
A person is usually alerted to brain cancer because of headache; as the tumor grows and presses against normal brain tissue, it causes pain. There are times, however, when a person with a brain tumor becomes nauseated, dizzy, or loses the sense of taste or smell. About a third of brain cancer patients have convulsions, the correct term for what are sometimes called seizures.

The diagnosis of brain cancer
When a brain tumor is suspected, the retina of the eye and the optic nerve are examined. X-rays are also taken. The CT scanner has made the diagnosis of brain tumors much simpler and is used whenever possible.

The treatment of brain cancer
The treatment for cancer of the brain is surgery or radiation therapy, and sometimes a combination of the two. Because of the blood-brain barrier, few chemicals injected into the bloodstream reach the brain; for this reason, chemotherapy is not frequently used to treat brain cancer.

A brain tumor, or as much of it as possible, will be surgically resected if it is accessible, whether it is cancerous or benign. Brain tumors are always dangerous, since there is no room for expansion inside the skull. A tumor presses against normal brain tissue and causes damage.

Radiation therapy is often used when a brain tumor cannot be entirely removed by surgery.

When chemotherapy is used, it is sometimes injected directly into the brain through a small, implanted tube. A relatively new group of anti-cancer drugs called nitrosoureas have been effective in some cases.

Bibliography

American Cancer Society. *Unproven Methods of Cancer Management*. New York: American Cancer Society, 1971.

Adams, D., & Deveau, E. *Coping with Childhood Cancer*. Reston, Virginia: Reston Publishing Co., 1984.

Brody, J., with Holleb, A. *You Can Fight Cancer and Win*. New York: McGraw-Hill, 1978.

Cameron, E., & Pauling, L. *Cancer and Vitamin C*. New York: Warner Books, 1981.

Furman, E. *A Child's Parent Dies*. New Haven: Yale University Press, 1974.

Glucksberg, H., & Singer, J. *Cancer Care*. New York: Scribner's, 1982.

Gonick, L., & Wheelis, M. *The Cartoon Guide to Genetics*. New York: Barnes and Noble Books, 1983.

Harsanyi, Z. & Hutton, R. *Genetic Prophecy: Beyond the Double Helix*. New York: Rawson Wade, 1981.

Jackson, E. *Telling a Child About Death*. New York: Hawthorne, 1965.

Koocher, G. & O'Malley, J. *The Damocles Syndrome*. New York: McGraw-Hill, 1981.

Kubler-Ross, E. *On Death and Dying*. New York: Macmillan, 1969.

————. *Questions and Answers on Death and Dying*. New York: Macmillan, 1974.

————. *To Live Until We Say Goodbye*. New York: Prentice-Hall, 1975.

Levitt, P. & Guralnick, E. *The Cancer Reference Book*. New York: Facts on File Inc., 1979.

MacDonald, J. *When Cancer Strikes*. Toronto: McClelland and Stewart, 1979.

Morra, M. & Potts, E. *Choices: Realistic Alternatives in Cancer Treatment*. New York: Avon, 1980.

Pendleton, E. *Too Old to Cry . . . Too Young to Die*. Nashville: Thomas Nelson, 1980.

Prescott, D. & Flexer, A. *Cancer: The Misguided Cell*. New York: Scribner's, 1982.

Rosenbaum, E. *Living with Cancer*. New York: Praeger, 1975.

Schiff, H. *The Bereaved Parent*. New York: Penguin, 1978.

Sontag, S. *Illness as Metaphor*. New York: Farrar, Straus & Giroux, 1978.

Terry, L. & Horn, D. *To Smoke or Not to Smoke*. New York: Lothrop, Lee and Shepard Co., 1969.

Thomas, L. *The Lives of a Cell: Notes of a Biology Watcher.* New York: Bantam, 1975.

Whelan, E. *Preventing Cancer.* New York: W.W. Norton, 1978.

Wolfe, A. *Helping Your Child to Understand Death.* New York: Child Study Association of America, 1958.

Index